Psychosocial Perspectives on Community Responses to Covid-19

This highly topical edited book documents the community response to Covid-19 across national contexts, exploring the widespread development and mobilisation of community initiatives and groups. It provides rich analysis of case studies from the Global North and South, including South Africa, the USA, India, China, Mexico, Brazil, Italy, Australia, the UK, Turkey, and Argentina.

The Covid-19 pandemic motivated a significant community response globally, with the widespread development and mobilisation of "bottom up" community initiatives and groups. These community responses were an essential yet often unseen and unrecognised means by which people survived the pandemic. This book asks questions such as how were community responses to Covid-19 shaped by national, cultural, and political processes and phenomena; how did community responses to Covid-19 interact with public policies, on health, education, and social welfare; and what are the likely political implications of the community response to Covid-19? Discussing the provision of abortion care in Latin America, the support to marginalized communities in Kolkata, and the mobilisation of carnival "krewes" in New Orleans, to give a few examples, the volume adopts and develops a novel socio-cultural psychological approach, weaving together contributions from scholars working in diverse disciplinary fields.

The volume highlights the importance of integrating multiple levels of analysis, including psychological, sociological, and political/ideological, to investigate how communities respond to crises such as the Covid-19 pandemic, and how they can plan for and manage future crises. It is essential reading for academics and students in psychology and the social sciences, as well as policy makers, charities, and third-sector organisations.

Emma O'Dwyer is a senior lecturer in political psychology at the University of Greenwich, London, UK. Her research interests include how people understand and orient towards issues like foreign policy and military intervention, and political participation, citizenship, and social change, examined frequently through the lens of social representations theory.

Luiz Gustavo Silva Souza is an associate professor in social psychology at Fluminense Federal University, Brazil. His research interests involve social representations, identities, and practices; ideology, active minorities, and mutual aid; the social-psychological understanding of health issues and contexts, action research, veganism, and human-animal relations.

Psychosocial Perspectives on Community Responses to Covid-19

Networks of Trust and Social Change

Edited by Emma O'Dwyer and
Luiz Gustavo Silva Souza

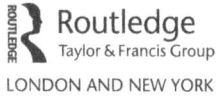
Routledge
Taylor & Francis Group

LONDON AND NEW YORK

Designed cover image: Getty

First published 2023
by Routledge
4 Park Square, Milton Park, Abingdon, Oxon OX14 4RN

and by Routledge
605 Third Avenue, New York, NY 10158

Routledge is an imprint of the Taylor & Francis Group, an informa business

British Library Cataloguing-in-Publication Data
A catalogue record for this book is available from the British Library

Library of Congress Cataloging-in-Publication Data
Names: O'Dwyer, Emma, editor. | Souza, Luiz Gustavo Silva, editor.
Title: Psychosocial perspectives on community responses to COVID-19 :
networks of trust and social change / edited by Emma O'Dwyer, Luiz
Gustavo Silva Souza.
Description: Abingdon, Oxon ; New York, NY : Routledge, 2023. |
Includes bibliographical references and index. |
Identifiers: LCCN 2022036738 (print) | LCCN 2022036739 (ebook) |
ISBN 9781032295060 (paperback) | ISBN 9781032295091 (hardback) |
ISBN 9781003301905 (ebook)
Subjects: LCSH: COVID-19 Pandemic, 2020---Political aspects--Case
studies. | COVID-19 Pandemic, 2020---Social aspects--Case studies. |
COVID-19 Pandemic, 2020---Psychological aspects--Case studies. |
Community organization--Case studies. | Political participation--Case
studies. | Social psychology--Case studies.
Classification: LCC RA644.C67 P792 2023 (print) | LCC RA644.C67
(ebook) | DDC 616.2/4144--dc23/eng/20221114
LC record available at https://lccn.loc.gov/2022036738
LC ebook record available at https://lccn.loc.gov/2022036739

ISBN: 978-1-032-29509-1 (hbk)
ISBN: 978-1-032-29506-0 (pbk)
ISBN: 978-1-003-30190-5 (ebk)

DOI: 10.4324/9781003301905

Typeset in Bembo
by MPS Limited, Dehradun

Contents

List of contributors   viii
Foreword   xiii
Acknowledgements   xvi

1 Social Distance and Social Connection: A Psychosocial
   Approach to the Community Responses to Covid-19   1
   LUIZ GUSTAVO SILVA SOUZA AND EMMA O'DWYER

PART I
Psychosocial and Psychological Resources to the
Community Response to Covid-19   13

2 The Role of Emotions in Grassroots Activism in
   Mexico City   15
   TOMMASO GRAVANTE AND ALICE POMA

3 Resilience, Organisation, Engagement: Defying
   Inequalities in Carrying Out Community Work in
   Rio de Janeiro's Favelas During the Covid-19 Pandemic   27
   LUANA ALMEIDA DE CARVALHO FERNANDES, ALFREDO ASSUNÇÃO, AND
   PEDRO PAULO GASTALHO DE BICALHO

4 Volunteering Motivation to Combat Covid-19: Evidence
   from Community Responses in China   37
   SUSAN SCHWARZ, GARY SCHWARZ, AND QING MIAO

5   Grassroots Movements and Covid-19 in Buenos Aires.
    Vital Networking and Social Media in Times of Crisis   51
    VICTORIA D'HERS

6   Collective Action, Protest, and Covid-19 Restrictions:
    Offline and Online Community Participation in
    Italy and Australia   66
    CARLO PISTONI, MAURA POZZI, EMMA F. THOMAS, AND
    CRAIG MCGARTY

7   How can Covid Mutual Aid Groups be Sustained Over
    Time? The UK Experience   79
    JOHN DRURY, MARIA FERNANDES-JESUS, GUANLAN MAO,
    EVANGELOS NTONTIS, ROTEM PERACH, AND DANIEL MIRANDA

PART II
**Communities Transforming Social Representations
and Public Policies**   91

8   Reimagining Infrastructure of Care in the Pandemic Time:
    Sketches from Kolkata   93
    RAKTIM RAY, AMIT CHATTERJEE, KOUMI DUTTA, AND
    DANA SOUSA LIMBU

9   Abortion Care in Times of Crisis: An Autonomous
    Feminist Model in Latin America and the Caribbean   107
    MARIANA PRANDINI ASSIS, ORIANA LÓPEZ URIBE,
    RUTH ZURBRIGGEN, AND VERÓNICA VERA

10 Clash of Cultures: Bureaucracy Meets Localism,
    Informality, and Trust in Responding to the Covid-19
    Crisis in Cape Town   119
    MANYA VAN RYNEVELD, ELEANOR WHYLE, AND LEANNE BRADY

11 Psychological, social, and political implications of UK
    Covid-19 mutual aid groups   133
    EMMA O'DWYER AND LUIZ GUSTAVO SILVA SOUZA

12 Re-Constructing the Meaning of Aid through the
Politicisation of Communities in a Welfare State:
The Psychological Responses to the Governmental
Aid Plans against Covid-19 in Turkey   145
S. BENGISU AKKURT, AHMET ÇOYMAK, AND YASIN KOÇ

13 Covid-19, Carnival, and Community in New Orleans, 2020   157
MARTHA RADICE

Index   170

Contributors

Sümeyra Bengisu Akkurt has a Bachelor's degree from Istanbul Şehir University and a Master's from Kadir Has University, Turkey. She is a research assistant at Abdullah Gül University and her research interests in social psychology include social identities, prejudice, and discrimination, collective action, and prosocial behavior.

Mariana Prandini Assis is an assistant professor of political science at the Federal University of Goiás, Brazil. Her research focuses on feminist political and legal theory, social movements, informality, and law and politics.

Alfredo Assunção is a professor in psychology at Universidade do Estado do Rio de Janeiro, Brazil and has visiting positions at the Universidade Eduardo Mondlani (Mozambique) and at Fundação Oswaldo Cruz, working at the Centre for the Studies on Tobacco and Health of the National Public Health School Sérgio Arouca.

Amit Chatterjee is an associate professor at the Department of Geography at Sidho-Kanho-Birsha University (SKBU), India. Amit has successfully completed a number of collaborative research and consultancy projects, including those on urban co-benefits (UNU, Japan) and politics of care in pandemic time (UCL, UK).

Pedro Paulo Gastalho de Bicalho is a specialist in legal psychology and an associate professor at the Psychology Institute of the Federal University of Rio de Janeiro, Brazil. He is also a visiting professor at Eduardo Mondlane University (Mozambique), San Carlos University (Guatemala), and the Republic University (Uruguay).

Leanne Brady works as an embedded researcher in Emergency Medical Services (EMS), the Western Cape Government's public ambulance service in South Africa, and is completing a PhD in Health Policy and Systems Research. She was involved in a Covid-19 mutual aid network – Cape Town Together – and a mobile vaccination initiative known as the Vaxi Taxi.

Ahmet Çoymak is a transnational peace activist and peace psychologist. He is currently affiliated with and the founder of the School of Psychology at Abdullah Gul University, Turkey. His primary interests include the content of the social self, gender relationships, civic engagement, political trust, stereotyping, and prejudice.

Victoria D'hers is a professor at the University of Buenos Aires, and National University of La Plata, Argentina, and an adjunct researcher at the National Council for Scientific and Technical Research of Argentina, and the Centre for Sociological Research and Studies. Her research interests include sociology of body/emotions, and environmental sociology.

John Drury is a professor of social psychology at the University of Sussex, UK. He has been studying the psychology of and behaviour in crowd events for nearly 30 years – including in emergencies and disasters, protests and social movements, religious festivals, music, and sports events.

Koumi Dutta completed a Ph.D in preventative and social health and is presently associated with a premier medical college of Kolkata, India. Koumi has worked as a volunteer for Quarantined Students Youth Network from its inception. Her research interest is in epidemiological studies related with health and physiological behaviour.

Luana Almeida de Carvalho Fernandes has a background in social psychology and is currently an environmental, social, and corporate governance analyst at the Federation of Industry of Rio de Janeiro, Brazil and a member of the Childhood and Youth Axis.

Maria Fernandes-Jesus is a lecturer at York St John University (UK) and an associate researcher at the Centre for Social Research and Intervention (CIS-Iscte, Portugal). Her research interests broadly relate to collective action, participation, and climate justice, particularly how communities resist and overcome social injustice and power inequalities.

Tommaso Gravante is a researcher at the Interdisciplinary Research Centre on Sciences and Humanities (CEIICH), UNAM, Mexico. His main research interests concern the role of emotion in protest and social movements, and the biographic consequence of protest.

Yasin Koç (he, him) is an assistant professor of social psychology at the University of Groningen, Netherlands. His main research interests include privilege acknowledgment, multiple conflicting identities, coping with stigma, and experiences of and reactions to emancipation.

Oriana López Uribe is a pansexual feminist from Mexico and holds a degree in ocial communication from UAM-Xochimilco. Her expertise on sexual and reproductive justice is focused on narrative change, access to education, and health services.

Guanlan Mao is a research assistant for the Groups and Covid project at the University of Sussex, UK. He will begin a doctorate in clinical psychology at the University of Oxford in September 2022.

Craig McGarty is a social and political psychologist whose work focuses on intergroup relations, collective action, intergroup relations, online activism, and stereotyping. McGarty has worked previously at the Australian National University, Murdoch University and Western Sydney University and is now transitioning to a late career role as an independent researcher.

Qing Miao is a professor of management in the School of Public Affairs at Zhejiang University. China. He is also the Chief Expert of the Academy of Social Governance of Zhejiang University. His research interests include social enterprise, charity management, corporate social responsibility, and leadership in the public sector.

Daniel Miranda is an assistant research professor at the Measurement Center MIDE UC, Pontificia Universidad Católica de Chile and an associate researcher at the Center for Studies of Conflict and Social Cohesion. His research interests include the intergenerational transmission of political inequality, political socialization, and youth political participation.

Evangelos Ntontis is currently a lecturer in social psychology at the School of Psychology and Counselling at the Open University, UK. His research focuses on collective responses to disasters and extreme events, as well as on social movements, leadership, and mass mobilisation.

Emma O'Dwyer is a senior lecturer in political psychology at the University of Greenwich, London, UK. Her research interests including how people understand and orient towards issues like foreign policy and military intervention, and political participation, citizenship, and social change, examined frequently through the lens of social representations theory.

Rotem Perach is an applied social psychology researcher whose research interests include facemasks, disinformation, solidarity, and culture. Previously, Rotem worked as a postdoctoral researcher at Goldsmiths, University of London, UK and at the University of Sussex, UK. Currently, he is a senior research fellow in the University of Westminster, UK.

Carlo Pistoni is a lecturer in social and community psychology at the Catholic University of Milan and Brescia, Italy, and a researcher associated with the Research Centre on Community Development and Organisational Quality of Life (Brescia). His research interests concern social and community participation in its various forms.

Alice Poma is a full-time researcher at the Social Research Institute of the National Autonomous University of Mexico (IIS-UNAM), and a teacher in the postgraduate programs in Sustainability Sciences and Political and

Social Sciences at UNAM. Her main lines of research are emotions, social movements and socio-environmental, and climate activism.

Maura Pozzi is an associate professor in Social and Community Psychology at the Catholic University of Milan, Italy. Her research interests concern different forms of participation. She is co-investigator in several research on social action: from volunteerism, to blood donation, to collective action, including social movements, and political participation.

Martha Radice is a social anthropologist whose work focuses on the social, spatial, and cultural dynamics of cities. Martha is an associate professor in the Department of Sociology and Social Anthropology at Dalhousie University, Halifax, Canada, and is a past president of the Canadian Anthropology Society.

Raktim Ray is currently a lecturer at the Development Planning Unit, UCL, UK. His research interests lie at the intersection of development studies and urban geography. His current research focuses on two themes: politics of care and infrastructure for spatial occupation.

Gary Schwarz is a professor in public management and strategy and director of the Public Management and Regulation Group at Queen Mary University of London, UK. His research focuses on how organisations and individuals can improve their performance, innovation, and leadership.

Susan Schwarz is an assistant professor at King's College, London, UK and Deputy Director of the MSc programme in the Strategy, International Management, and Entrepreneurship group. Her research focuses on the role of "capitals" – human capital, social capital, financial capital, and psychological capital – and their impact on individual and organisational outcomes.

Dana Sousa-Limbu holds a Master's in social development practice from the Bartlett Development Planning Unit at UCL, UK and is currently a graduate teaching assistant and events officer there. Dana's research interests include exploring postcolonial perspectives on the ways in which people express themselves, their identities, and ethnicities.

Luiz Gustavo Silva Souza is an associate professor in social psychology at Fluminense Federal University, Brazil. His research interests involve social representations, identities, and practices; ideology, active minorities, and mutual aid; the social-psychological understanding of health issues and contexts, especially in primary health care; action research, veganism, and human-animal relations.

Emma Thomas is a professor of psychology at Flinders University, Australia. Her work sits at the nexus of social and political psychology and focusses on understanding when, why, and how people commit to engaging in action to bring about social change for disadvantaged groups in society.

Manya van Ryneveld is a PhD candidate at the University of the Western Cape, South Africa. Her research examines localised, community health system responses to health crises through the lens of gender and care work, using the Covid-19 pandemic and the HIV/AIDS epidemic in South Africa as case studies.

Verónica Vera is a feminist social communicator and a founding member of Las Comadres, an activist network that accompanies women and other people in their abortions in Ecuador.

Eleanor Whyle is a researcher in the health policy and systems division at the University of Cape Town, South Africa and is currently completing a PhD on social values and health system reform. Eleanor also worked closely with a Cape Town-based community-led rapid response to the Covid-19 pandemic.

Ruth Zurbriggen is an activist and researcher at the Feminist Collective La Revuelta and Socorristas en Red-Feministas que Abortamos, in Argentina, who has been accompanying people in their abortions for over 12 years. With a specialization in gender studies, Ruth focuses on pedagogy and sexual education in public education institutions.

Foreword

During the Covid-19 pandemic, people around the world mobilised in their communities to help themselves and other people to survive the severe hardships which the crisis brought. They set up community groups, organised with their neighbours to provide practical and financial assistance, as well as vital social support. Often, this outpouring of "mutual aid" exposed chronic inequalities as well as the underfunding of essential public services. This volume explores the ways in which communities from both the Global North and South responded to the pandemic, drawing upon diverse case studies of community action and solidarity during the crisis. The chapters are also rich in terms of the different disciplinary, theoretical, and methodological approaches which are adopted.

Our aim with this volume is to integrate these different perspectives to forward a psychosocial understanding of the community responses to Covid-19. In Chapter 1 (Souza & O'Dwyer, 2022), we sketch out such a potential approach, drawing upon work in the social representations and active minorities traditions of our discipline — social psychology. We do not attempt to make a case for the primacy of our approach over the multiple, fascinating disciplinary and theoretical perspectives offered in the volume, but instead suggest it as one potentially useful analytical lens with which to interpret the subsequent chapters.

The volume is dvided into two sections. Section 1 – *Psychosocial and psychological resources to the community response to Covid-19* – comprises six chapters, each of which document and analyse individual and collective resources mobilised in community responses such as emotions, motivation, moral convictions, narratives, social identities, personal and group efficacy. The first chapter in this section (Gravante & Poma, 2022) focuses on Mexico City and analyses the ways in which two specific mutual aid groups there – CDMX Ayuda Mutua (Mexico City Mutual Aid) and Huerto Roma Verde (Green Roma Garden) – through their prefigurative practices, troubled hegemonic neoliberal emotions and offered possibilities for resistance. Following on from this, Chapter 3 (Fernandes et al., 2022) provides a window into the community response to Covid-19 in the Rio de Janeiro favelas by analysing the perspective of one instrumental and influential community organiser named Rogéria. Chapter 4 (Schwarz et al., 2022) draws upon work on the psychology of volunteering and emergency management to analyse volunteering and non-profit organisations in China during Covid-19, and addresses the question of volunteering motivation using mixed-methods. Adopting a more sociological approach, Chapter 5 (D'Hers, 2022) focuses on the intersection of Covid-19, exclusion, and inequality with an analysis of a publication and social media network created to counter negative attitudes and stereotypes about slumdwellers – La Garganta Poderosa. Methodologically, this chapter makes use of digital ethnography and participant observation in assemblies and women's meetings during 2021, in a neighbourhood in Buenos Aires. Chapter 6 (Pistoni et al., 2022) offers a useful perspective on the community response to Covid-19, by providing a social psychological analysis of predictors of online and offline collective action in two contexts – Italy and Australia. Concluding this section, Chapter 7 (Drury et al., 2022) provide a further social psychological analysis of the experiences of participants in Covid-19 mutual aid groups in the United Kingdom, particularly focusing on the role of social identity processes.

In the six chapters which comprise Section 2 – *Communities transforming social representations and public policies* – there is sustained attention to the ways in which the community response to Covid-19 engaged with and responded to the state and public policies, and how it critiqued the current political order and offered alternatives. Chapter 8 (Ray et al., 2022) draws on ethnographic fieldwork focusing on the Quarantined Student-Youth Network (QSYN) in Kolkata, India, to elaborate how the politics of care is operationalised through solidarity networks and conceptualises solidarity networks as an invisible form of infrastructure, providing an invaluable rejoinder to current conceptualisations of infrastructure in postcolonial contexts. Following this, Chapter 9 (Assis et al., 2022) highlights the work of Red Compañera, a Latin American and Caribbean network of organisations and feminist/lesbofeminist collectives that accompany women, girls, and other people to have abortions with care and in safety. Here, the authors discuss the challenges they encountered as members of Red Compañera during the pandemic, and through this, propose a feminist abortion accompaniment model of care which is a direct critique and alternative to the status quo. Then, in Chapter 10 (Van Ryneweld et al., 2022) the work of community action networks in South Africa is described, with a specific focus on Cape Town Together. The chapter describes the vital actions taken by this group and offers a discussion of the challenges and possibilities present in integrating community-led responses such as these with state responses to public health emergencies. In Chapter 11 (O'Dwyer & Souza, 2022), a further discussion of UK Covid-19 mutual aid groups is provided, paying particular attention to the psychological and political implications of these groups and what this might mean for future social and political change. Continuing the focus on political processes, Chapter 12 (Akkurt et al., 2022) analyses the community response to Covid-19 in Turkey, constructing it as a battleground between the authoritarian national government, and the liberal municipal authorities and citizens which spearheaded these initiatives. Finally, Chapter 13 (Radice, 2022) provides a digital ethnography of the ways in which carnival "krewes" in New Orleans, USA, pivoted to maintain a sense of community and provide social support, solidarity, and other assistance to the local community during the pandemic.

Taken together, the chapters highlight the importance of integrating *multiple* levels of analysis – psychological, sociological, and political/ideological – to investigate how communities respond to crises such as the Covid-19 pandemic. We argue that such an integrative approach is necessary, as it forces us to step outside our disciplinary and theoretical silos in order to re-conceptualise, to pose alternative questions, and offer critique. We hope that this volume provokes these critical questions in some way.

We argue that each of the chapters included here demonstrates the almost inevitable capacity of people and groups to *respond* in a crisis. Detailed are case studies of groups and individuals responding to help their neighbours, the vulnerable and disadvantaged, in contexts which vary substantially in terms of political regime, inequality, and the processes of marginalisation and exclusion. Each of these case studies, we argue, functions as a rejoinder to prevailing narratives of public alienation, apathy, and political paralysis. We draw strength and hope from their creative prefiguration of a more just and equal future, necessary as we look ahead to a future of deeper crisis precipitated by climate change.

Acknowledgements

Many thanks to the following people, who provided invaluable support, guidance, or inspiration (or indeed, all three): Carl Cullinane, Arabella Atkinson, Chris Hewer, Rye Lane Mutual Aid, the SE15 Solidarity Fund, and Rhiannon Firth. Thanks also to the Quarantined Student-Youth Network for their permission to reproduce images included in this volume.

1 Social Distance and Social Connection: A Psychosocial Approach to the Community Responses to Covid-19

Luiz Gustavo Silva Souza and Emma O'Dwyer

Introduction

At the time of writing (May 2022), Covid-19 is no longer the biggest news. On the 24th of February 2022, Russia invaded Ukraine and war has been back to the centre stage of Europe. The world faces anxieties resembling those of the Cold War, the risk of the escalation of violence and total annihilation. The impression that history had achieved its final stability with the unquestioned supremacy of "liberal democracy" has decidedly faded away. History is back with full force and is wide open. In fact, instead of stopping, history seems to have gained increased speed. Giddens' (1990) "careering juggernaut"[1] seems to be accelerating near dangerous cliffs. The world accumulates global crises: the menace of world war, the environmental catastrophe caused by global warming, and the Covid-19 pandemic. Unlike the downfall of relatively isolated civilisations of previous eras, the possible collapse of the current interconnected global civilisation may signify the collapse of humanity (Diamond, 2005).

Vaccination against Covid-19 is now protecting large parts of the population worldwide. However, the emergence of vaccine-resistant SARS-CoV-2 variants remains a possibility, as well as the advent of new pandemics. The horrific exploitation of non-human animals, especially in factory farming, is a time bomb in this regard (Paim & Alonso, 2020). These crises and the prospect of their dreadful consequences highlight the need to enhance our control of the "juggernaut", through political, social, cultural, institutional, and scientific activity. The human and social sciences can contribute insight into how to understand the origins and phenomenology of the catastrophes we face and how to manage their outcomes. One of our intellectual tasks is to understand these global crises from a psychosocial perspective.

This chapter outlines a psychosocial approach to the Covid-19 pandemic and the community responses to the crisis. We conceive psychosocial phenomena as distinct from and articulated with psychological and socio-cultural phenomena. In the kaleidoscope of the human and social sciences, psychosocial concepts form singular shapes and provide a particular way of regarding individuals, groups, and societies. They are not like attitudes, beliefs, or behaviours, for example, which may be conceptualised as the properties of individuals. Nor are

DOI: 10.4324/9781003301905-1

they like culture, political systems, or modes of production, for example, which pertain to societies[2]. Adopting a psychosocial approach involves conceptualising phenomena that are simultaneously individual and collective. This means focusing on how historical and socio-cultural phenomena are realised ("made real") in the daily experiences of individuals and groups, i.e., how collective forces shape subjective experiences. This also means considering how the actions of individuals or active minorities (Moscovici, 1976) transform groups, institutions, communities, and societies. Psychosocial analyses are thus inherently contextualised. The psychosocial approach proposed here is based on the concepts of social representations, social identity, and social practices[3].

Social Representations

Covid-19 is a respiratory disease caused by a virus, SARS-CoV-2 ("the coronavirus", as it became known). In March 2020, the World Health Organisation declared Covid-19 a pandemic. In technical-scientific terms, the description of the phenomenon is straightforward: a disease; a causal agent; a pandemic, which is a function of the interconnectedness of societies and the contagious properties of the virus. If modern societies were "scientific", as they are often perceived (Moscovici & Hewstone, 1983), these general terms would be sufficient for the construction of knowledge about Covid-19. Every society, institution, community, group, and individual would readily accept the scientific explanation about the existence of the virus and its action in the human body; the need for systematic experiments to validate treatments, medications, and vaccines; and the behavioural measures necessary to mitigate the damage. The cognitions about Covid-19 would be almost homogeneous and all alternative views would be cast aside as superstition.

This is, obviously, far from reality. Modern societies, groups, and individuals do not merely repeat the scientific discourse. More generally, they do not *perceive* but *construct* the relevant social objects by applying a substantial amount of creativity and combining knowledge coming from numerous and heterogeneous sources, such as common sense, tradition, family and group norms, philosophy, religion, morality, the law, the media, the arts, i.e., a complex fabric of knowledge in which science is only one of the threads (Bangerter, 1995; Jovchelovitch, 2008; Moscovici & Hewstone, 1983). That is, they construct social representations, a set of articulated images, beliefs, and attitudes that correspond to the very reality of the object they perceive, and which contribute to guiding their practices and reinforcing their identity (Jodelet, 1999).

Many reasons make these representations "social". The most immediate one is the fact that they are shared. Individuals and groups, sometimes separated by great distances of time and space, believe the same ideas, evoke the same images, and experience the same emotions when dealing with a certain object. However, there are stronger reasons: First, these representations are social because they have been constructed throughout history and consolidated in culture, i.e., they are at least in part a collective-coercive object in a

Durkheimian sense. Based in language, they are simultaneously a product and source of the shared symbolic and imaginary cultural structures. Second, they have religious-like properties. Individuals and groups adhere to social representations through cognitive-emotional patterns resembling "faith". Consonant with the classical Durkheimian definition of religion (Durkheim, 1912/1995), social representations unite the adherents into a community[4]. Finally, they are social because of their contextual-communicative nature. Individuals and groups (re)construct social representations through interaction, dialogue, and shared practices. In this sense, thinking, perceiving, remembering, feeling, and behaving are not functions of an individual and their brain but truly shared activities. Social representations are a way to see the psychosocial nature of psychological processes.

Worldwide, individuals and groups have fervently adhered to conspiracy theories as parts of theories of common sense[5] to explain Covid-19 and guide their practices. We highlight examples from the USA, the UK, and Brazil, but these processes have been common in many countries. In the USA, highly influential politicians and large populational groups have endorsed the ideas that the virus was intentionally manufactured by China, the pandemic was a hoax or a strategy of social control, and the health measures were an attack on individual freedom. Some individuals believed that the recently installed telecommunication masts transmitting 5G internet waves created the coronavirus, which led them to destroy many of these masts by arson (Jolley & Paterson, 2020). American individuals endorsing conspiracy theories tended to exhibit lower levels of adherence to health-protective measures (Bierwiaczonek et al., 2020). In a sample composed mainly of Americans and Britons, individualists tended to express lower intentions to adhere to restrictive health measures such as social distancing whereas collectivist individuals tended to report greater endorsement of these measures (Biddlestone et al., 2020).

In Brazil, as in other countries, two different ways of representing Covid-19, as a "health crisis" or an "economic crisis", have been fuelling social conflict. Individuals and groups that anchored[6] Covid-19 as an "economic crisis" believed that the country should not follow restrictive health measures because of the associated damage to employment and the economy. They believed that Covid-19 was nothing more than a "little flu" and that the mainstream media and health authorities were exaggerating the seriousness of the disease as well as the numbers of infections and deaths (Justo et al., 2020). In extrapolations typical of common sense, some of them believed that Covid-19 is a left-wing disease created by a communist country (China); that Brazil should be protected from communists; that this must be achieved by a strong virile positioning in the social arena, associated with the belief that "we are strong and do not need to use masks or practice social distancing", and so on (Morel, 2021). These ideas are in line with the science-denialist and sexist views of the far-right Brazilian politicians that have been gaining increasing prominence in the federal, state, and municipal government spheres. The supporters of these politicians make them person–symbols (icons) of their social representations[7].

At the beginning of the pandemic, we investigated the theories of common sense constructed by Brazilian middle-class individuals about Covid-19 (Souza et al., 2021). We found that our participants represented Covid-19 as a dramatic disease that attacks those with low immunity. They conceived immunity as an individual property cultivated through maturity, mental strength, and moral correctness. In their representations, Covid-19 was also a crisis that would ultimately improve humankind, forcing people to abandon individualism, consumerism, and hedonism (e.g., the abuse of alcohol, bars, drugs, and sex), and cherish values of family life, respect for authority, and obedience to God. These representations have clear ideological (pro-dominance) properties since they contribute to concealing and naturalising the social inequalities that have been causing the greater Covid-19 vulnerability of the working classes and minorities (in Brazil and elsewhere). They produce ideology from the bottom-up through the creativity of embodied and contextualised social thought.

Thus, conceiving Covid-19 became much more than understanding concepts about a respiratory disease. The representations of Covid-19 included conspiracy theories but were not limited to them. Indeed, these representations go beyond the belief that certain actors are secretly planning to control others or impose harm. In some cases, representing Covid-19 became a fierce defence of Western individualism and way of life, family values, morality, capitalism against communism, and so on. Perceiving a new disease and pandemic became a platform to defend social representations in their wider sense, i.e., a worldview, a cosmology.[8] Observing the level of emotional and behavioural involvement in this process, one may say that individuals and groups worship their representations–cosmologies with "religious fervour" and that these representations form and unite communities. A circularity binds the two terms: one can conceptualise social representations as those beliefs/attitudes that unite a community, and a community as that group united by particular social representations. More specifically, a community may be defined as a group of people who share social representations, identity, and the conditions of access to power (both in its symbolic and material aspects) (Campbell & Jovchelovitch, 2000).[9]

A psychosocial analysis of our time must consider the advent and popularisation of the internet and social media. Indeed, these technical innovations have produced a substantial increase in the interconnectedness of individuals, groups, societies, and a further acceleration of modernity's "careering juggernaut". Websites and social media platforms became central public arenas where individuals and groups engage in interaction, communication, dialogue, struggle, and violence, i.e., central arenas of production of social representations. The problem is again one of social connection and trust.[10] Who should we trust when sources of social influence clash? Impersonal scientific authorities like the World Health Organisation and Ministries of Health or our family, group of friends, like-minded colleagues, and community?

Interaction in the social media arenas has important characteristics that favour trust in the ingroup to the detriment of impersonal specialised authorities. It intensifies the contact among individuals, the spread of ideas, consensual beliefs and images, the emotional appeal of communication (attention-grabbing, simplified, and fast) to the detriment of its rational aspects, and the personification of social representations in heroes and mortal enemies, sacred and demonic figures (Consentino, 2020). Social media thus mobilises powerful psychological forces towards the strengthening of ingroups (sometimes called "bubbles") and exclusion of outgroups, and they do so in part to favour the economic interests of giant social media corporations (Justo et al., 2020). If history is characterised by the alternation of dominance between rationally focused dialogue and an emotionally focused cult of authority, as crowd psychology suggests (Moscovici, 1985), the dynamics of social media seem to be favouring the latter. Different public arenas have been producing different social representations. Social representations are the symbolic environment we live in. Thus, conflicting social groups are effectively, at least in part, living in different worlds.

Social Identities

A psychosocial approach must look beyond the idea that theories of common sense lack logic or scientific rigour and consider their functions and effects. Theories of common sense allow individuals and groups to grasp an object, tame it and drain it of the menace of the unknown. With them, social actors guide and justify their practices and construct and reinforce social identities. Social identity is at the heart of social representations since, as discussed above, belonging, adherence, community-making, and faith in a common reality are central features of social representations.

The social representations of Covid-19, like those of diseases in general, favour the process of othering. Individuals and groups go to great psychological-practical lengths to affirm that the disease has nothing to do with themselves or their groups. In the social representations they mobilise, the disease typically originates from others (outgroups), and the others are its preferential or sole victims (Eicher & Bangerter, 2015; Joffe, 1995; Souza et al., 2021). This othering process articulates fundamental functions of social representations and social identities: they make familiar the unfamiliar whilst protecting the ingroup and fulfilling identity motives including self-esteem. At the basis of social identity lies the ingrained necessities of constructing and maintaining positive emotions and cognitions regarding the self and simplifying the social world through categorisation and stereotypes. Considering the phylogenetic-adaptative advantages of such processes, it is not unreasonable to consider that they are invariants of the human condition. However, "all the rest must incorporate an historical analysis" (Hogg & Abrams, 1998, p. 16). A psychosocial approach to social identities considers that categories and stereotypes are socio-historically constructed and assimilated through socialisation (Tajfel, 1969). As socio-historical processes, they are hard to shift, but also open to change. The concept of social identity places the group inside the self, providing insight into the inherently intertwined individual-collective nature of human experience.

Social representations and social identities may act as dangerous forces leading individuals and groups to health risks, social discrimination, and harmful inter-group relations. However, they may also be the psychosocial resources necessary to fight a pandemic, empower a minority group and overcome inequality. As Howarth (2006) states, the process of (re)construction of social representations may allow groups and communities to challenge violence and stigmas. Social identities may be the way for groups and individuals to make sense of challenging conditions, acquire agency, and receive support, constituting a "social cure" (Jetten et al., 2017). This highlights the need to consider how social representations and social identities are effectively enacted in particular contexts and how they relate to social hierarchies and domination.

Worldwide, individuals and groups constructed social identities to respond to the pandemic. Gravante and Poma (Chapter 2 in this volume) argue that grassroots activities in Mexico helped individuals convert feelings of guilt into efficacy; the self-perception as a "careless person who got Covid-19" into that of an activist fighting a political-economic system that imposed the heavier burden of Covid-19 on marginalised groups. Likewise, Pistoni et al. (Chapter 6 in this volume), examining experiences of online protest in Italy and Australia, demonstrate how social identification is crucial for social mobilisation and collective action. Similarly, Drury et al. (Chapter 7 in this volume) show that the construction of social identities in British mutual aid groups provided the participants with the perception of social support and a sense of empowerment, ultimately enhancing well-being during the difficult time of the pandemic. In Turkey also, Akkurt et al. (Chapter 12 in this volume) highlight that political social identification was a crucial feature of many community responses. And in New Orleans, Radice (Chapter 13 in this volume) reveals how social clubs producing carnival helped individuals to build the sense of community necessary to fight the pandemic. In a very human way, the menace is socially symbolically constructed, and the cure is also psychosocial.

Social Practices

The rapid and global spread of information about Covid-19 created the pandemic and the coronavirus as a quasi-universal symbol and the sense that the crisis has been affecting the whole world. In most countries, these powerful beliefs have been accompanied by a substantial change in daily life, with the lockdowns, mask-wearing, and other substantial changes in social practices. A reified object (the coronavirus) has entered the public sphere and provoked the urgent need for theories of common sense (Souza et al., 2021). For some individuals and groups, it has also created a sense of urgency about the need to act not only to protect oneself from illness and death but also other people living in the same street, ward, slum, village …, i.e., in the same geographical and/or symbolic world. In many cases, these actors produced communities where they did not exist, creating new identities, social representations, and means of exerting power. They have formed networks of trust and social change.

These events have had some characteristics of "social big bangs" (Moscovici, 1988/2005) albeit different in size. In such conditions, the naturalised and seemingly immovable social reality is shaken and acquires remarkable fluidity. The social actors involved are animated by new energy and regain the status of makers of history. They construct strong bonds of loyalty and commitment to moral action transforming the institutionalised *status quo* into institutionalising action. The external conditions of the pandemic and the community responses may have made new practices seem irreversible possibly leading to radical changes in social representations (Flament, 1994). Social representations and social practices have different ways of determining each other. Social representations provide the symbolic environment in which social practices occur. Social practices, in turn, reinforce, modify, or totally transform social representations (Rouquette, 2000).

Social practices are, thus, socially defined sets of behaviours that may become, on the other hand, definers of the social. If social representations turn the unfamiliar familiar, social practices in their behavioural polyphasia have the capacity to turn the familiar unfamiliar. Like social representations are characterised by cognitive polyphasia, social practices are characterised by *behavioural* polyphasia. Social representations make the past "more real than the present" (Moscovici, 1984, p. 10) whereas social practices, on the other hand, may place social actors into the transformative possibilities of the present. Thus, an artist may "discover" part of their sculptural work in the marble itself; an educator in the very act of teaching may "be led" to a new teaching technique; a word or a gesture from a patient may prompt a medical doctor to adapt a treatment protocol, and so on. Every time social practices are enacted, the internal-external "here and now" forces may transform these practices. These transformations may gain collective force in a group, institution, or community, and lead to substantial modifications of social representations. We define behavioural polyphasia as the multiple sources of behaviour determination (body, movement, emotion, context, and interactions) with which an individual engages to act in the present. Since its symbolic-material configurations are always singular, behavioural polyphasia is a constant generator of novelty in practices and representations. This concept may be a fruitful addition to a theory interested in social change like the theory of social representations.

Facing the Covid-19 pandemic, communities reacted to a crisis that has been threatening their physical and symbolic existence. They have been doing so in a world structured by social, economic, and political inequality, and in societies founded on intergroup struggles. In the international arena and particular nation-states, dominant groups and organisations have been oppressing a large majority of the world population, imposing poverty, violence, hunger, sexual exploitation, environmental devastation, exploitative work conditions, state brutality, and war. Therefore, Covid-19 has been an additional crisis in a worldwide reality characterised by ongoing human and environmental catastrophes (Preston & Firth, 2020). The community responses are not something new. While dominant groups use their material and symbolic power to keep their privileges, marginalised communities have always been reacting to this state of affairs, applying individual and collective creativity and efficacy to resist oppression and create spaces of expression and participation (Campbell & Jovchelovitch, 2000; Freire, 1968/2013).

The widespread functionalist perspective on social influence (Moscovici, 1976) depicts communities as passive entities that would be mostly dependent on the elites and the state to react to a crisis like the Covid-19 pandemic. Moscovici's (1976) distinction between the functionalist and genetic models of social influence provides useful guidance here. From the functionalist perspective, social practices must ensure the smooth adaptation of individuals to a pre-existing social reality, stable institutions, and norms. Deviance is represented as a pathology and conceived as the lack of information, resources, and capacity to exert social influence. In this model, social interventions aim to improve the functionality of society and the adaptation of marginalised groups. Society is conceived as a system in equilibrium. The model highlights the importance of leaders, i.e., individuals capable of embodying the prevalent social norms and assimilating minorities into them.

In contrast, the genetic model on social influence, which we adopt in this book, depicts individuals and groups as active agents in the construction of their social environments and society. Deviance may represent a positive challenge to normality, which is actively posed by individuals, groups, and society itself. Marginalised groups, minorities, are also seen as a permanent source of social influence. Therefore, social interventions must consider the practices, representations, values, identities, and norms held by marginalised groups in the process of creating new practices and transforming social realities. Innovation is as important as conformity. This perspective conceives society as a field of conflict, a place of battle among different worldviews, projects, and practices. This genetic view on social influence clarifies the shift from charity to solidarity, enacted by many mutual aid groups (Chevée, 2021). Solidarity involves fully considering the voices of the marginalised groups, their desires and projects for the construction of social reality.

Individuals and groups involved in the community responses to Covid-19 have constituted active minorities, effectively creating communities and challenging prevalent contemporary values, such as egoism and competition, and the dependence upon the state to conduct social intervention. Furthermore, it is important to highlight the instances in which they acted as counter-ideological active minorities, directly or indirectly denouncing and fighting oppression. Ideology is the way(s) "in which meaning serves to establish and sustain relations of domination" (Thompson, 1990, p. 56). In challenging prevalent social and cultural structures, active minorities do not necessarily challenge ideology. Indeed, some active minorities are overtly ideological in that they support, for example, racism, classism, and sexism. Furthermore, minorities that fight against certain kinds of oppression may consistently or at times reinforce others (Davis, 1981/2019, for example, showed that the American White feminist movement has often been racist). Social representations are not hegemonic or critical in themselves but in the way they are employed, in particular contexts, to defend particular interests (Howarth, 2006).

Globally, marginalised groups have been the most vulnerable to Covid-19. When communities protect them from Covid-19 and other threats, they (re) affirm these groups' very right to exist and thrive in a world order that is hegemonically indifferent to (or in favour of) their extermination (Preston & Firth, 2020). Communities have been creating spaces of cooperation and collective sense-making in cultural contexts typically characterised by strong individualism. They have been constructing active forms of citizenship in cultural contexts that reinforce the passive position of the individual regarding the state (O'Dwyer et al., 2022). They have been using social media to enable fast, flexible, efficient localised action and put local interests ahead of the interests of the "intangible" social media corporations. That is, they have been reconstructing social representations and social identities in ways that do not reinforce but indeed contest domination.

D'Hers (Chapter 5 in this volume) describes how a social movement in Argentina has been (re)constructing the narrative about the pandemic, challenging official, dominant, and ideological narratives. Likewise, Assis et al. (Chapter 9 in this volume) discuss how a Latin-American feminist network foregrounds the perspective, voice, and power of marginalised women, strongly grounded in the principle of "circularity" in knowledge-power relationships (the carers also receiving care from the public). They challenge utopia, highlighting the need to live the "desirable world" *in the present*, in the form of micro-contexts and relationships, promoting autonomy not as individualism but as the power that individuals acquire through an affective and effective network. In South Africa also, Van Ryneveld et al. (Chapter 10 in this volume) demonstrate how bottom-up responses to the pandemic have been effectively changing the application of public policies. These initiatives have been addressing focal issues such as Covid-19 prevention and food insecurity but also providing multiple possibilities to address gender violence, racism, and classism.

It is important to avoid romanticising the community responses or taking them as a panacea. To steer modernity's "careering juggernaut" in the right direction, the elites, institutions, corporations, and the national states must rise (and be led to rising) to the civilisational challenge of identifying with oppressed groups and their struggles. But such a project would not succeed without the effective participation of communities and counter-ideological active minorities. They are, in many cases, showing the path to overcome human oppression, the atrocities perpetrated against non-human animals, the environment, and indeed the whole planet. The chapters of this book pay homage to their energy and creativity.

Notes

1 Giddens (1990) proposes the image of a "careering juggernaut" (p. 53) to capture the experience of living in modernity. Individuals and organisations can control the juggernaut only to some extent; its path and pace are often unpredictable. The ride can be exhilarating and hopeful, but it can also lead to a terrible crash and complete destruction.

2 Psychology and sociology focus on a binary relation between an individual or collective actor and an object. On the other hand, social psychology produces its concepts and analyses focusing on a tripartite relation which includes the other (*alter*), i.e., it adopts a "psychosocial regard" (Moscovici, 1984/2008).

3 The chapters of this volume are based on different theoretical perspectives in Social Psychology, Sociology, and Anthropology. In this chapter, we do not intend to reduce this diversity into a single theoretical perspective but rather to provide one way (among many others) of articulating the different concepts and phenomena to which they refer.

4 Moscovici (1988/2005) refers to this property of social representations in radical terms: "By saying that in an idea a power exists that operates like a physical energy we do not mean the term to be taken metaphorically. On the contrary, by it we define the substratum without which we are nothing to one another. Without it there is no chance of lasting social bonds being forged" (p. 114).

5 In this chapter, we use the terms "social representations" and "theories of common sense" interchangeably. However, the word "theory" should not be taken in its scientific sense. Social representations include contradictory, irrational, and unconscious aspects.

6 Anchoring and objectification are the psychosocial mechanisms used to construct social representations (Moscovici, 1961, 2000). They are the processes of classifying objects into social and group categories and norms (anchoring) and finding or creating images capable of making ideas concrete and visible in the "real world" (objectification). Finding categories and images is a simultaneously individual and collective activity, i.e., it is "social" in the broad terms outlined above.

7 The personification of knowledge may be a part of the objectification mechanism operating in the construction of social representations (Moscovici & Hewstone, 1983). This process has clear connections with crowd psychology. Charismatic leaders seek to embody social representations to exert their effects on the crowds (Moscovici, 1985).

8 It is possible to say that Moscovici (1988/2005), for example when discussing Weber's "spirit of capitalism", describes social representations as cosmologies including an ethos: "[What would be the spirit of capitalism?] Being neither a theological doctrine nor an economic method nor an institution, it is indeed a social representation, neither more or less" (p. 182).

9 *En passant*, we note that communities differ from what group psychologists refer to as the "small group" (defined by its interconnectedness) because they do not necessarily share spatial and temporal constants and awareness of all its members.

10 Modernity is characterised by the absence of an ultimate source of authority, leading to permanent conflicts between competing claims for authority (Giddens, 1990). In conditions of modernity, the traditional sacred versus profane domains have been replaced by human-centred domains of representations and practices, i.e., the reified and consensual universes (Moscovici, 2000).

References

Bangerter, A. (1995). Rethinking the relation between science and common sense: A comment on the current state of SR theory. *Papers on Social Representations*, *4*(1), 1–18. https://psr.iscte-iul.pt/index.php/PSR/article/view/191

Biddlestone, M., Green, R., & Douglas, K.M. (2020). Cultural orientation, power, belief in conspiracy theories, and intentions to reduce the spread of Covid-19. *British Journal of Social Psychology, 59*, 663–673. 10.1111/bjso.12397

Bierwiaczonek, K., Kunst, J.R., & Pich, O. (2020). Belief in COVID-19 conspiracy theories reduces social distancing over time. *Applied Psychology: Health and Well-Being, 12*(4), 1270–1285. 10.1111/aphw.12223

Campbell, C., & Jovchelovitch, S. (2000). Health, community and development: Towards a social psychology of participation. *Journal of Community & Applied Social Psychology, 10*, 255–270. 10.1002/1099-1298(200007/08)10:4<255::AID-CASP582>3.0.CO;2-M

Chevée, A. (2021). Mutual aid in north London during the Covid-19 pandemic. *Social Movement Studies, 21*(4), 413–419. 10.1080/14742837.2021.1890574

Consentino, G. (2020). *Social media and the post-truth world order. The global dynamics of disinformation.* Palgrave Macmillan. 10.1007/978-3-030-43005-4

Davis, A.Y. (1981/2019). *Women, race & class.* Penguin.

Diamond, J. (2005). *Collapse. How societies choose to fail or succeed.* Penguin.

Durkheim, E. (1912/1995). *The elementary forms of religious life.* The Free Press.

Eicher, V., & Bangerter, A. (2015). Social representations of infectious diseases. In G. Sammut, E. Andreouli, G. Gaskell, & J. Valsiner (Eds.), *The Cambridge handbook of social representations* (pp. 385–396). Cambridge University Press.

Flament, C. (1994). Structure, dynamique et transformation des représentations sociales [Structure, dynamics, and transformation of social representations]. In J.C. Abric (Ed.), *Pratiques sociales et représentations* (pp. 37–58). PUF.

Freire, P. (1968/2013). *Pedagogia do oprimido [The pedagogy of the oppressed].* Paz e Terra.

Giddens, A. (1990). *The consequences of modernity.* Polity Press.

Hogg, M.A., & Abrams, D. (1998). *Social identitifications. A social psychology of intergroup relations and group processes.* Routledge.

Howarth, C. (2006). A social representation is not a quiet thing: Exploring the critical potential of social representations theory. *British Journal of Social Psychology, 45*(1), 65–86. 10.1348/014466605X43777

Jetten, J., Haslam, A., Cruwys, T., Greenway, K.H., Haslam, C., & Steffens, N.K. (2017). Advancing the social identity approach to health and well-being: Progressing the social cure research agenda. *European Journal of Social Psychology, 47*, 789–802. 10.1002/ejsp.2333

Jodelet, D. (1999). Représentations sociales: un domaine en expansion [Social representations: an expanding domain]. In D. Jodelet (Ed.), *Les représentations sociales* (pp. 47–77). PUF.

Joffe, H. (1995). Social representations of AIDS: Towards encompassing issues of power. *Papers on Social Representations, 4*, 29–40. https://psr.iscte-iul.pt/index.php/PSR/article/view/200/164

Jolley, D., & Paterson, J.L. (2020). Pylons ablaze: Examining the role of 5G COVID-19 conspiracy beliefs and support for violence. *British Journal of Social Psychology, 59*, 628–640. 10.1111/bjso.12394

Jovchelovitch, S. (2008). The rehabilitation of common sense: Social representations, science and cognitive polyphasia. *Journal for the Theory of Social Behaviour, 38*, 431–448. 10.1111/j.1468-5914.2008.00378.x

Justo, A.M., Bousfield, A.B.S., Giacomozzi, A.I., & Camargo, B.V. (2020). Communication, social representations and prevention – Information polarization on COVID-19 in Brazil. *Papers on Social Representations, 29*(2), 4.1–4.18. https://psr.iscte-iul.pt/index.php/PSR/article/view/533

Morel, A.P.M. (2021). Negacionismo da Covid-19 e educação popular em saúde: para além da necropolítica [Covid-19 denialism and the popular education approach to health: Going beyond necropolitics]. *Trabalho, Educação e Saúde, 19*, e00315147. 10.1590/1981-7746-sol00315

Moscovici, S. (1961). *La psychanalyse, son image et son public. Étude sur la représentation sociale de la psychanalyse* [*Psychoanalysis: Its image and its public. Study on the social representation of psychoanalysis*]. PUF.

Moscovici, S. (1976). *Social influence and social change*. London: Academic Press.

Moscovici, S. (1984/2008). Introduction. Le domaine de la psychologie sociale [Introduction. The domain of social psychology]. In S. Moscovici (Ed.), *Psychologie sociale* (pp. 5–22). PUF.

Moscovici, S. (1984). The phenomenon of social representations. In R.M. Farr & S. Moscovici (Eds.), *Social representations* (pp. 3–69). Cambridge University Press.

Moscovici, S. (1985). *L'âge des foules. Un traité historique de psychologie des masses* [*The age of the crowd: A historical treatise on mass psychology*]. Complexe.

Moscovici, S. (1988/2005). *The invention of society. Psychological explanations for social phenomena*. Polity Press.

Moscovici, S. (2000). *Social representations. Explorations in social psychology*. Polity Press.

Moscovici, S., & Hewstone, M. (1983). Social representations and social explanations: From the 'naive' to the amateur scientist. In M. Hewstone (Ed.), *Attribution theory: Social and functional extensions* (pp. 98–125). Blackwell.

O'Dwyer, E., Souza, L.G.S., & Beascoechea-Seguí, N. (2022). Rehearsing post-Covid-19 citizenship: Social representations of UK Covid-19 mutual aid. *British Journal of Social Psychology* .*61*(4), 1245–1262. 10.1111/bjso.12535

Paim, C.S., & Alonso, W.J. (2020). *Pandemics, global health and consumer choices*. Cria.

Preston, J., & Firth, R. (2020). *Coronavirus, class and mutual aid in the United Kingdom*. Palgrave Macmillan.

Rouquette, M.L. (2000). Paradoxes de la représentation et de l'action: des conjonctions sans coordination [Paradoxes of representation and action: conjunctions without coordination]. *Les Dossiers des Sciences de l'Éducation, 4*, 17–22. 10.3406/dsedu.2000.930

Souza, L.G.S., O'Dwyer, E., Coutinho, S.M.S., Chaudhuri, S., Rocha, L.L., & Souza, L.P. (2021). Social representations and ideology: Theories of common sense about COVID-19 among middle-class Brazilians and their ideological implications. *Journal of Social and Political Psychology, 9*(1), 105–122. 10.5964/jspp.6069

Tajfel, H. (1969). Cognitive aspects of prejudice. *Journal of Biosocial Science, 1*(S1), 173–191. 10.1017/S0021932000023336

Thompson, J.B. (1990). *Ideology and modern culture. Critical social theory in the era of mass communication*. Polity.

Part I

Psychosocial and Psychological Resources to the Community Response to COVID-19

2 The Role of Emotions in Grassroots Activism in Mexico City

Tommaso Gravante and Alice Poma

Introduction

The chapter analyses experiences of grassroots groups that have organised themselves in Mexico City since the Covid-19 outbreak, using mutual aid and solidarity to respond to the needs of the most vulnerable people. These self-managed groups and networks have worked, among other things, on making and delivering food and baskets with basic products, setting up community kitchens, offering medicines, providing psychological support to cope with the pandemic and increased domestic violence resulting from the lockdown, as well as supporting children's education and even forging creative alliances to facilitate the exchange of services or sale of products made by professional artisans and local farmers. The hypothesis that we consider in this chapter forwards that the social impact of these mutually supported communities is not limited to addressing the social needs the pandemic caused, but also involves prefigurative political practices. By analysing the politicisation process of the trauma experienced by those affected by the pandemic and the collectivisation of certain emotions, such as pain, shame, guilt, and powerlessness, among others, we show how these groups are proposing practices, emotions and "feeling rules" (Hochschild, 1975) antagonistic to those promoted by the neoliberal model, such as individualism, egoism, competitiveness, narcissism, contempt for the poor, etc. The analysis of the emotional dimension of these experiences will be conducted based on Hochschild's sociological theory of emotions as sociocultural constructs and the literature on emotions and protest (Jasper, 2018). Among the case studies, we have identified *CDMX Ayuda Mutua* (Mexico City Mutual Aid), a new grassroots group, and the ongoing work of organisations already in place – such as *Huerto Roma Verde* – which we have followed since March 2020 using qualitative research techniques, such as online observation, surveys, and interviews.

Emotions and Political Action: A Sociological Approach

Emotions are a determining part of the political arena insofar as they participate in all its processes, such as the emergence of certain political actors, the

DOI: 10.4324/9781003301905-3

choice of strategies, the radicalisation of narratives, the construction of collective identity and burnout, among others. The research presented in this chapter is based on a sociological perspective with a sociocultural approach.

Talking about emotions as a sociocultural construct means considering the cultural context in which the individual feeling is inserted, i.e., their experience, culture, social interactions, biography, and, of course, their historical moment. The starting point of this approach, which goes beyond the classical view of emotions as a foundational part of irrationality, as shown also by psychological constructivist theories (see Feldman Barrett, 2017), is the proposal of American sociologist Arlie Hochschild (1975, 1979, 1983), which is characterised by two aspects. First, unlike classical psychology, which considers emotions as individual and biological internal states, Hochschild believes that emotions are a sociocultural construct and therefore changeable according to the social context and historical period, thus overcoming the organicist and universal view of emotions. Second, the individual is considered a conscious and active being in relation to their emotions, i.e., people are not only able to perform superficially by manifesting the most appropriate emotions in accordance with the situation (Goffman, 1959), but can reflect on what they feel, managing their emotions, evoking, suppressing (Hochschild, 1979, 1983), or channelling them (Gould, 2009) to adapt or defy the society's feeling rules.

The concept of feeling rules developed by Hochschild (1975) refers to the social norms that determine what emotion one should feel on each occasion and with what intensity and duration. Human beings follow these rules to fit into society, and they can be as simple as expressing grief at a funeral and joy at a wedding, or much more complex, involving a political dimension. In this case, there are certain feeling rules, such as loving one's country, which can be linked to an ideology, to certain values or political beliefs. Therefore, all social, economic, and political systems, in addition to promoting and legitimising a series of norms or structural rules of social, legal, and economic discipline, are also characterised by a series of feeling rules necessary to consolidate the dominant system (Hochschild, 1975).

We define these norms as "dominant" feeling rules. For example, in the current pro-industrial capitalist system, a feeling rule identified by Hochschild (2016) is loyalty to companies, even when they are responsible for polluting territories, with all the consequences this entails for ecosystems and human health.

Moreover, Hochschild shows that feeling rules also follow patterns of gender, class, and race. In this case, it is necessary to look at the direction of the "ideal" emotion – according to the cultural system. For example, admiration for authority figures or people in the higher social classes can be promoted on the one hand, while contempt for certain categories of people such as the incarcerated, the homeless, migrants, etc. is promoted on the other.

When these rules are not observed, they provide for the application of social penalties such as verbal reproach, distancing, exclusion, mockery, or social stigma. To act in accordance with the feeling rules, and therefore reduce the disharmony between what is felt (the real emotion) and what society tells us we should feel in each situation (the ideal emotion), and thus avoid social penalties, Hochschild developed the concept of emotional management or emotional work. Management can be superficial, when the "ideal" emotion is only expressed, or deep, when the subject comes to actually feel it. Like any rule, feeling rules can be respected, as happens in most of our daily lives, but they can also be challenged. Social movements as agents of social change can challenge not only some dominant feeling rules, but also consolidate their "antagonistic" rules, which over time can come to shape their own emotional culture (Taylor & Rupp, 2002).

Hochschild's proposal broke with the rationality vs. emotion dichotomy since the emotional processes described are also characterised by including cognitive processes. In other words, we feel about what we think, and we think about what we feel. The split in Cartesian dualism between emotions and rationality was also reflected in Jasper (1997) when he stated that "emotions are closely connected with the cognitive meanings one constructs about the world, and to the moral valuations accompanying them. Such links are present even when emotions are in conflict with moral and cognitive knowledge" (p. 110), and when he introduced the concept of thinking-feeling processes (Jasper, 2018). Hochschild's (1979) proposal directly links the micro to the macro dimension of politics, emphasising that "elites, and indeed social groups in general, struggle to assert the legitimacy of their framing rules and their feeling rules. Not simply the evocation of emotion but laws governing it can become, in varying degrees, the arena of political struggle" (p. 568).

This perspective has been applied in the field of study of social movements, protest, and grassroots activism. Jasper's (2018) theory of action also shares this approach, and further provides a typology of emotions characterised by the durability of their cognitive processing and their temporality. Therefore, we can identify emotions that are generated from limited cognitive processing – such as quick automatic responses to events and information – among which the author includes reflex emotions and urges, and emotions with high cognitive processing such as affective commitments and moral emotions, which are longer lasting and built based on people's culture and biography (Jasper, 2018, p. 13).

These typologies are particularly useful when identifying what a person feels, first because human feelings are characterised by the presence of several emotions at the same time, but also because we are not always able to express what we feel clearly, or we do so using different terms. Jasper's constructivist approach focuses on understanding the context and the elements that influence the construction of emotions rather than the words they are named after. This has also made it possible to identify how we can find very different emotions under the same word. For example, the fear of being late for a work meeting is not the same as the fear of getting sick or dying from Covid-19, or the fear of losing one's home and being displaced due to war.

Finally, in view of what we present below, it is also important to highlight the relationship between emotions and political practices. Emotions and action are inseparable, just as emotion and cognition are inseparable. Emotions guide action, but emotions are also generated from action to the point where it is possible to develop attachments to certain practices or tactics. The pre-figurative practices carried out by the grassroots groups analysed in this chapter are characterised by a close coherence between means and ends, between values and objectives. Thus, we show that certain practices, such as mutual support in the case of the pandemic, are characterised by certain emotions, such as love and compassion, which make it possible to manage the guilt, vulnerability, loneliness, and social stigma experienced by many people who became ill with Covid-19, especially among the working classes.

Method

Since March 2020, because of the health and social emergency caused by the Covid-19 pandemic, different forms of political activism have emerged, mainly focused on addressing the demands of everyday life and promoting solidarity in communities and social groups – usually urban – affected by the pandemic and neglected by the state. Since the beginning of the pandemic, the world has witnessed the activities of thousands of mutual support groups and networks. Some of them are born from previous experiences, which have transformed their agendas due to the social crisis caused by the pandemic. Other groups have formed in response to health and social emergencies. Just to give an idea of the social phenomenon discussed in this text, following our previous research (Gravante & Poma, 2022; Gravante, 2022), more than 4,000 groups were registered in the United Kingdom, more than 300 in the United States as of April 2020, and around 188 groups in 57 cities in Spain in March 2020 alone. In the same way, hundreds of soup kitchens were created in the cities of Mexico, Chile, Argentina, Uruguay, Italy, and Greece, i.e., organised spaces in poor suburbs where food was collected and cooked for the neediest (Leetoy & Gravante, 2021). Based on these data, a first categorisation of grassroots activism during the Covid-19 pandemic was carried out, system-atising these experiences in terms of their practices, organisation, and values (Gravante, 2022).

Subsequently, based on these results, we carried out a qualitative investigation of two experiences that have arisen in Mexico City, the findings of which will be presented in turn. The two groups are quite heterogeneous. The first, *CDMX Ayuda Mutua* (Mexico City Mutual Aid), is a group formed in March 2020 to support people who found themselves with health or economic problems be-cause of the pandemic. The main activity of the group, made up of about 20 permanent members, has been to collect basic goods through donations orga-nised into food baskets and distributed to struggling families. Since March 2020, the group has donated more than 2,000 baskets to the needy. In addition, they have organised creative and cultural activities to support artists and artisans in the city, such as virtual art galleries, raffles, courses, and online workshops. At the time of writing (April 2022), the collective is still active. Its activities are focused on supporting people and artists in need in the city and other grassroots experiences such as feminist, LGTBQ, or migrant support collectives.

The second group is *Huerto Roma Verde* (HRV), which arose in 2012 from a citizen initiative and civil society organisations with the objective of recovering for the community a public space that was abandoned and deteriorating. It is currently one of the only occupied community spaces in the city. Its members define HRV as a biosocial laboratory where projects related to the environment and sustainability are developed. The group is also an active player in the Mexican climate movement. With the pandemic, HRV activists also adjusted their agenda by creating mutual support network projects to support those most in need.

We monitored and collected data from these two groups from March 2020 to December 2021. To understand the role of emotions in their practices, we conducted semi-structured individual interviews and focus groups with members of both groups and a closed-ended survey with 16 *CDMX Ayuda Mutua* activists as a newly formed group. We had more knowledge of the *Huerto Verde Roma* activists as we had been following them since 2018 due to their involvement in climate activism. Finally, we triangulated the qualitative data with data from a national survey on the impact of the pandemic on Mexican grassroots activism that the authors conducted in July and August 2021 ($N = 105$).

The Role of Emotions in Grassroots Activism During the Pandemic

Ever since the social crisis due to the pandemic was brewing, different social responses have been emerging from different social actors, ranging from denial and minimisation of the risks of the disease, indifference, concern for the economy, panic, and cynicism, to solidarity and mutual support. The responses of many countries' political elites, such as the USA (Trump), Brazil (Bolsonaro), the UK (Johnson), and Mexico (López Obrador), were characterised by a series of statements that emphasised denial and minimisation of the disease's risks, cynicism, legitimisation of social determinism, and acts of racism and discrimination towards Asian or migrant communities, strengthening the stigma towards Covid-19 patients (Gravante & Poma, 2022). For example, in Mexico, as in many other countries, the discourse of the political and entrepreneurial elites on the pandemic was characterised by underestimation, denial, cynicism, individualism, and economic functionalism, among other things (Gravante & Poma, 2022). For example, at the end of March 2020 the President repeatedly stated "Don't stop going out. I'm going to tell you when you don't go out", and the workers of Grupo Salinas, owned by the entrepreneur Roberto Salinas Pliego, were forced to work despite the high rate of infections and deaths. The lockdown was not as mandatory or restricted as in other countries such as Italy, and most poor people (around 60% of the population) could not stay at home, because they worked informally. Most people stayed at home for a time, relying on savings or even getting into debt, and they were badly affected. The inability of the state to ensure the right of citizens to stay at home with a salary or financial support in a context of extreme inequality, together with the cynicism of part of the business and upper classes, the shortcomings of the health system, as well as the high rates of obesity and comorbidities, has led Mexico to the highest mortality rates of Covid-19 in the world.

All these practices, positions, and statements contributed to breaking the social fabric of communities deeply hit by the social effects of the pandemic, driving a process of social polarisation that spawned conflicts between those who followed the health measures and those who did not; those who got sick or were vulnerable and those who were not; or those who could stay at home and those who could not. This polarisation feeds the process of *othering of the disease threat*, that is, the construction of a representation of a particular out-group and the association of that representation to the cause of a disease (Eicher & Bangerter, 2015). While in the US the out-groups were the Black or Chinese people, in Mexico they were the poorest, who could not stay at home. People who got sick were identified as guilty, and those who died as weak, while those who could stay at home and did not get sick became the virtuous (Gravante & Poma, 2022; Poma, 2022).

On the other hand, around the world we saw the creation of networks of mutual support and solidarity focused on supporting the neediest throughout the pandemic. The grassroots activism that emerged in these months was characterised mainly by the practice of direct social action in everyday life. Direct social action is characterised by ignoring the traditional repertoire of contentious action directed against institutional authorities or powerful social actors, insofar as it is a practice aimed at improving the human condition within a given group or community. Through this direct action, activists aim to change society through the politics of everyday life in which the boundaries between public and private spheres are blurred (Bosi & Zamponi, 2015).

The social responses to the Covid-19 crisis from grassroots activism are directly linked to a series of emotions that the different groups legitimise, evoke, strengthen, and collectivise. The process of collectivisation of emotions is the main strategy used by the collectives and is very important in a context such as the pandemic, where people's isolation has worsened, with the resulting difficulty in sharing and expressing their feelings. To this we must add the individualistic character of the neoliberal model, which blames people for their discomfort, going so far – in the context of the pandemic – as to consider the citizen who does not get sick as virtuous, and blame the one who does, without considering each person's different circumstances.

The result is that, on the one hand, people directly affected by the virus or who lost a loved one to it experience the disease or their bereavement as an individual matter, characterised by guilt and stigma. On the other hand, vulnerable people such as seniors living alone and in need of help feel undervalued as they are no longer "productive", or some of them were not asking for support because they were ashamed of showing a lack of self-sufficiency. In these cases, like with immigrants or people who have lost their economic independence because of the pandemic, the dominant feeling rules cause shame and guilt in those who are struggling, a process that generates even more helplessness and powerlessness in the face of Covid-19 and its social consequences.

Political Impacts of the Emotions of Trauma and Resistance

Solidarity from grassroots groups has made it possible to overcome feelings of guilt and stigma thanks to a process of collective framing that allows the management of the emotions of trauma based on the emotions of resistance (Whittier, 2001).

From our data, in the case of the Covid-19 pandemic, the emotions associated with trauma, for example, are grief due to the loss of loved ones; fear, anguish, or anxiety about becoming ill or contagious; worry or anxiety about economic insecurity; shame about being vulnerable or becoming ill; helplessness in the face of the disease; and sadness due to isolation and collective suffering. To manage these unpleasant emotions, grassroots groups have promoted collective strategies that have had different political impacts in a micro social dimension.

One of the strategies we have already mentioned is to collectivise grief, which continues to be done through tributes to deceased activists, for example. In terms of fear management, one strategy is to facilitate contact with physicians and nurses who can support and advise in case of illness, as well as provide medicines to families who cannot afford them. In addition, many professionals such as yoga teachers, sports coaches, and psychologists offered free online workshops through the channels of the collectives. Campaigns by activists to promote local and artisanal consumption served to address the anguish resulting from the lack of employment, especially among informal workers who account for half of Mexico's productive workforce. Some people managed powerlessness by participating in these initiatives. In fact, the groups promoted the participation of people who were not physically vulnerable, so that they not only donated goods or received the aid, but also became active subjects.

The feeling rule that links the disease with shame and guilt – such as believing it to be divine punishment and the result of immoral behaviour (Eicher & Bangerter, 2015), or a consequence of personal characteristics instead of social structures and inequalities (Souza et al., 2021) – was challenged by these groups by sharing messages on their social networks such as "Having Covid is neither a crime nor a sin. Don't discriminate, don't judge, don't disclose. Support the person who suffers from it. Tomorrow, it could be you".

Breaking with the individualisation of blame for getting sick has also made it possible to politicise the pandemic as a consequence of the capitalist system, and to identify culprits, both among the political authorities and in economic power. Redirecting blame has made it possible to construct a political discourse around trauma and to politically frame the experience of suffering (Champagne, 1996; Whittier, 2001).

Another process that we emphasise from our research involves the so-called emotions of resistance (Whittier, 2001), such as hope, moral anger, indignation, pride, and reciprocal emotions such as love or respect, which are felt when organising, and which help to cope with the emotions of trauma and to generate emotional energy, among other things (Collins, 2001, 2012; Jasper, 2011, 2018). These emotions enable people affected by the pandemic to manage the pain, sadness, and fear and to overcome powerlessness and feelings of helplessness and vulnerability (Champagne, 1996; Whittier, 2001; Gravante, 2020). Evoking the emotions of resistance through the practices of grassroots groups has empowered many people to overcome powerlessness and create a framework of injustice (Gamson, 1992) around their situation of social vulnerability, as analysed in the case of women victims of violence (Poma & Gravante, 2019).

One consequence of this emotional work is that the people to whom the aid was directed became empowered and participated in the project. In this case, emotions such as guilt and shame for being sick or asking for help are transformed into compassion towards the most affected and pride for helping them.

This could be observed in the soup kitchens in the poorest outskirts of several cities, as well as in projects such as *Ayuda Mutua CDMX*, where some beneficiaries of the food baskets have become actively involved in the project by helping to distribute the baskets to other people and families and by supporting other projects.

By generating feelings of empowerment (Drury & Reicher, 2009), the emotions of resistance go beyond the event itself, impacting people's lives in the present and most likely in the future as they engage in new projects (Drury & Reicher, 2009), as we have seen among the people who have been involved in the documented experiences.

Furthermore, emotional work plays an important role in the construction of the antagonistic feeling rules based on compassion and solidarity, which counters the hegemonic feeling rules based on individualism and cynicism, as the activists of the *Ayuda Mutua CDMX* state: "Everyone deserves to feed their families and stay safe. We will get through this together".

The Construction of "Us" vs. "Them": Emotions and Collective Identity

Both emotions and feeling rules play an important role in the construction of collective identity, i.e., the construction of an "us" opposed to a "them" (Polletta & Jasper 2001; Bayard de Volo, 2006; Flesher Fominaya, 2010; Poma & Gravante, 2018). From this perspective, we define collective identity as "an individual, cognitive, moral and emotional connection to a wider community, category, practice or institution" (Polletta & Jasper, 2001, p. 285).

Among the emotions that play a central role in the construction of collective identity are not only reciprocal emotions (Jasper, 1997), i.e., those that group activists and participants feel towards each other, but also the emotions that group members feel towards their opponents (Bayard de Volo, 2006). Moreover, emotions towards opponents provide insight into the types of organisations and strategies that collectives choose, such as the decision of many grassroots groups not to collaborate with the government, political parties, or NGOs, favouring horizontal and informal relations with other groups.

What we were able to observe by monitoring the Mexican groups is that they managed to construct a collective identity that people affected by the pandemic could identify with and feel less alone. Collectivising the experience of the disease (we can all get sick, all of us are vulnerable) or the affectation of the crisis (we are living a bad time) is a strategy to make people feel part of a community under attack, which helps to overcome the individualisation of the vulnerability that characterises the neoliberal system and individualism. The construction of this "us" is based on the perception of a shared sense of injustice that is fuelled, on the one hand, by historical grievances such as inequality and structural poverty in the country, and on the other hand, by biographical grievances, such as the appalling working and housing conditions, especially in the suburbs, and the lack of access to hospitals, medicines, and education. This framework of injustice that characterises collective identity strengthens shared emotions (Jasper, 1997), i.e., the common emotions that activists and participants feel towards their adversaries or allies, such as resentment towards the government for not having created a decent free healthcare system accessible to all, or moral emotions such as indignation or outrage at the lack of care for the most vulnerable people, or compassion and solidarity towards other projects of mutual support. These circles of "us" and "them" are not static constructions, but dynamic, changing over time and because of activism. The widening of the "us" is due to the presence in the collectives studied of new social actors in the urban fabric, such as the collectives emerging from the recent wave of Latin American feminism and climate activism, anti-speciesist groups, LGTBQI+ collectives, libertarian groups and others. Thanks to the widening of the "us", grassroots groups are also changing, becoming not only initiatives that collect and distribute food and basic products, but also social laboratories where relationships based on compassion and solidarity are experienced in contrast to the neoliberal culture based on contempt and cynicism.

The emotional management that accompanies the practices of grassroots groups in the times of the pandemic, in addition to favouring the process of identification among participants, allows for the radicalisation of the political narrative, which we have observed in slogans such as "Capital is the virus", "Solidarity not charity" or "The best vaccine is organisation". We can therefore conclude that practices with a prefigurative character (Yates, 2014), such as horizontal organisation, decisions made by consensus, mutual support, respect for differences, among others, cannot be separated from the emotional culture of groups (Taylor & Rupp, 2002), which is shaped by experience in direct action, and which in turn also influences collective identity.

Conclusions

In this chapter, we have analysed the role of emotions in the activism that has emerged during these two years of health and social emergency through the experience of two mutual support groups in Mexico City.

Through a process of collectivisation of certain emotions, grassroots activism in times of Covid-19 has made it possible to manage the emotions that define the dominant cultural model (and the feeling rules behind it). This dominant model is characterised by the logic of losers vs. winners, which, legitimising social Darwinism, has created an emotional culture around illness (not only for Covid-19) where emotions such as shame and guilt, on the one hand, and selfishness and cynicism on the other, prevail. Managing these emotions associated with the experience of the pandemic, which we have defined as "trauma", as well as the emotions generated in direct action, defined as "resistance", has allowed for a process of politicisation of the lived experience, which has been framed as a social injustice. At the same time, it has allowed the emergence of antagonistic feeling rules based on feelings of compassion and solidarity.

Another salient finding is that emotions play a central role in the construction of participants' collective identity, which, on the one hand, has made it possible to overcome what Hochschild calls the empathy wall (Hochschild, 2016) – such as between people from different social classes who have not fallen into the narrative of the "virtuous" versus the "spreader" – and on the other, to widen the circle of an "us" affected by the pandemic.

Finally, we would like to highlight that the grassroots activism that has emerged throughout this crisis in Mexico City, as in other parts of the world, has made it possible to reinterpret the limits that confined the concept of care, generally conceived as an individualistic and gendered practice. In these experiences, care (and self-care) is framed as a collective responsibility, which is reflected in the activists' sayings: "self-care is political" and "care is revolutionary". Likewise, their protest posters show messages such as: "whatever you are doing, do it with your heart", or "weapon of mass reconstruction" with the image of a heart-shaped grenade.

References

Bayard de Volo, L. (2006). The dynamics of emotion and activism: Grief, gender, and collective identity in revolutionary Nicaragua. *Mobilization: An International Journal, 11*, 461–474. DOI: 10.17813/maiq.11.4.q21r3432561l21t7

Bosi, L. & Zamponi, L. (2015). Direct social actions and economic crises: The relationship between forms of action and socio-economic context in Italy. *Partecipanzione e Conflitto, 8*, 367–391. DOI: 10.1285/i20356609v8i2p367

Champagne, R. (1996). *The politics of survivorship.* New York: New York University Press.

Collins, R. (2001). Social movements and the focus of emotional attention. In Goodwin, J., James, J.M., & Polletta, F. (Eds.), *Passionate Politics: Emotions and Social Movements* (pp. 27–44). Chicago: University of Chicago Press.

Collins, R. (2012). C-escalation and D-escalation: A theory of the time-dynamics of conflict. *American Sociological Review, 77*, 1–20. DOI: 10.1177/0003122411428221

Drury, J., & Reicher, S.D. (2009). Collective psychological empowerment as a model of social change: Researching crowds and power. *Journal of Social Issues, 65*, 707–726. DOI: 10.1111/j.1540-4560.2009.01622.x

Eicher, V., & Bangerter, A. (2015). Social representations of infectious diseases. In Sammut, G., Andreouli, E., Gaskell, G., & Valsiner, J. (Eds.), *The Cambridge Handbook of Social Representations* (pp. 385–396). Cambridge, United Kingdom: Cambridge University Press.

Feldman Barrett, L. (2017). *How emotions are made: The secret life of the brain.* New York: Houghton Mifflin Harcourt.

Flesher Fominaya, C. (2010). Collective identity in social movements: Central concepts and debates. *Sociology Compass, 4*, 393–404. DOI: 10.1111/j.1751-9020.2010.00287.x

Gamson, W. (1992). *Talking politics.* Cambridge: Cambridge University Press.

Goffman, E. (1959). *Presentation of self in everyday life.* Garden City, NY: Doubleday.

Gould, D. (2009). *Moving politics: Emotion and ACT UP's fight against AIDS.* Chicago: University of Chicago Press.

Gravante, T. (2022). El activismo de base en tiempos de pandemia: Una primera caracterización cualitativa. In Gravante, T., Regalado, J., & Poma, A. (Eds.), *Viralizar la esperanza en la ciudad. Alternativas, resistencias y autocuidado colectivo frente a la covid-19 y a la crisis socioambiental,* (pp. 187–207). Mexico City: CEIICH-UNAM.

Gravante, T. (2020). Forced disappearance as a collective cultural trauma in the Ayotzinapa movement. *Latin American Perspectives, 47*, 87–102. DOI: 10.1177/0094582X20951773

Gravante, T., & Poma, A., (2022). How are emotions about COVID-19 impacting society? The role of the political elite and grassroots activism. *International Journal of Sociology and Social Policy, 42* (3/4), 369–383. DOI: 10.1108/IJSSP-07-2020-0325

Hochschild, A.R. (1975). The sociology of feeling and emotion: Selected possibilities. In Millman, M. & Moss Kanter (Eds.), *Another voice* (pp. 280–307). New York: Anchor.

Hochschild, A.R. (1983). *The managed heart. Commercialization of human feeling.* Berkeley, CA: University of California Press.

Hochschild, A.R. (1979). Emotion work, feeling rules, and social structure. *American Journal of Sociology, 85*, 551–575. DOI: 10.1086/227049

Hochschild, A.R. (2016). *Stranger in their own land: Anger and mourning on the American right.* New York: New Press.

Jasper, J.M. (1997). *The art moral of protest: Culture, biography, and creativity in social movements.* Chicago: University Chicago Press.

Jasper, J.M. (2011). Emotions and social movements: Twenty years of theory and research. *Annual Review of Sociology, 37*, 285–303. DOI: 10.1146/annurev-soc-081309-150015

Jasper, J.M. (2018). *The emotions of protest.* Chicago: University of Chicago Press.

Leetoy, S., & Gravante, T. (2021). Feeding solidarity and care. The grassroots experiences of Latin American soup kitchens in times of global pandemic. In Montoya, M.A., Rehner, J., Krstikj, A., & Lemus-Delgado, D., (Eds.), *COVID-19 and cities - Experiences, responses, and uncertainties* (pp. 147–160). Switzerland: Springer Nature. DOI: 10.1007/978-3-030-84134-8

Polletta, F. & Jasper, J.M. (2001). Collective identity and social movements. *Annual Review of Sociology, 27*, 283–305. DOI: 10.1146/annurev.soc.27.1.283

Poma, A. (2022). Emociones y polarización social en tiempo de Covid-19. In Hansberg Torres, O.E. (Ed.), *La vida emocional en la pandemia* (pp. 15–37). Mexico City: UNAM.

Poma, A. & Gravante, T. (2019). 'Nunca seremos las mismas de antes'. Emociones y empoderamiento colectivo en los movimientos sociales: el Colectivo Mujer Nueva (Oaxaca, México). *Desafíos, 31*(2), 231–265. DOI: 10.12804/revistas.urosario.edu.co/desafios/a.7308

Poma, A. & Gravante, T. (2018). Manejo emocional y acción colectiva: las emociones en la arena de la lucha política. *Estudio Sociológico, 36*, 593–616. DOI: 10.24201/es.2018v36n108.1612

Souza, L.G.S., O'Dwyer, E., Coutinho, S.M., Dos, S., Chaudhuri, S., Rocha, L.L., & Souza, L. P. de. (2021). Social representations and ideology: Theories of common sense about COVID-19 among middle-class brazilians and their ideological implications. *Journal of Social and Political Psychology, 9*(1), 105–122. DOI: 10.5964/jspp.6069

Taylor, V. & Rupp, L. (2002). Loving internationalism: The emotion culture of transnational women's organizations, 1888-1945. *Mobilization, 7*(2), 125–144. DOI: 10.17813/maiq.7.2.fw3t5032xkq5l62h

Whittier, N. (2001). Emotional strategies: The collective reconstruction and display of oppositional emotions in the movement against child sexual abuse. In Goodwin, J., James, J.M., & Polletta, F. (Eds.), *Passionate politics: Emotions and social movements* (pp. 233–250). Chicago: University of Chicago Press.

Yates, L. (2014). Rethinking prefiguration: Alternatives, micropolitics and goals in social movements. *Social Movement Studies, 14*(1), 1–21. DOI: 10.1080/14742837.2013.870883

3 Resilience, Organisation, Engagement: Defying Inequalities in Carrying Out Community Work in Rio de Janeiro's Favelas During the Covid-19 Pandemic

Luana Almeida de Carvalho Fernandes,
Alfredo Assunção, and
Pedro Paulo Gastalho de Bicalho

Introduction

Recognising the effects of the coronavirus pandemic in Brazil has emphasised the consequences of social inequality and violations of human rights across the country. The response of the Federal Government to the pandemic illustrates a deathly policy adopted by the State – which the Cameroonian intellectual Achille Mbembe (2003) defines as necropolitics – and points to some of the challenges for the creation of a world where dignified life is a right for all and not a privilege for a few.

The present chapter discusses the importance of social organisation and collective engagement. These processes are exemplified by the impact of community actions developed in Rio de Janeiro by major social actors to mitigate the effects of the pandemic. Rio de Janeiro is the second most populous city in Brazil – currently with more than 6 million inhabitants – and the place of the first death attributable to coronavirus in the country. News about the Covid-19 outbreak started to emerge more frequently by the end of January 2020 in Brazil. Soon after, at the beginning of March, the spread of the virus was declared a health emergency at the international level by the World Health Organisation (WHO), and then a pandemic.

Brazil is the sixth most populous and the fifth largest country in the world. For the first 12 months of the pandemic, the actions taken by the Brazilian government were considered inadequate and inefficient due to the lack of energetic measures to fight the spread of the disease. This lack of action intensified the crisis in the Brazilian public health system – a system that has been, in recent years, constantly overwhelmed, and devalued by the Federal Government.

The study "Avoidable Deaths from Covid-19 in Brazil" (Oxfam, 2021) showed that, in the first year of the pandemic, 120,000 deaths could have been

DOI: 10.4324/9781003301905-4

avoided if preventive measures such as social distancing and restrictions on crowds had been adopted. In the absence of effective governmental action, there were 305,000 more deaths than what was expected in the first year. Considering the economic consequences of Covid-19, the number of people living in conditions of famine in the world has quintupled since March 2020. In Brazil, the percentage of the population living in extreme poverty rose from 4.5% to 12.8%, and 116 million people faced some level of food insecurity, of which almost 20 million suffered from starvation (OXFAM, 2021).

Since the approval of the constitutional amendment 95 in December 2016 (which froze investments in social areas), Brazil has suffered from an intensified depreciation of its health system, and the closing of hospital beds and entire hospital facilities across the country. Many would consider this fact alone to be a sign of societal collapse. Many cities adopted lockdown and social isolation measures, while many of its citizens were not able to stop working. As stated by the Bolivian psychologist María Galindo (2020): in Latin America, the coronavirus exposes the colonial order of the world, pointing out that "here, the death sentence was written before Covid arrived on a tourist airplane" (p. 124). In the early months of the pandemic, the wealthiest were already affirming that the worst was over, regardless of the growing number of deaths among the poorest, who suffered from the difficulties of getting access to any basic treatment.

The consequences of the coronavirus in the slums of Rio de Janeiro point to social inequality as a structural feature of Brazilian society. A glance at the spread of cases of infection and deaths reveals the multiplicity of ways of existence that share the urban context. It indicates that in many of these scenarios, access to decent housing, drinking water, and minimum income is increasingly distant from the recommendations of international health agencies. In Brazil, the consequences of the pandemic reveal not only income differences across social groups. Through an intersectional analysis that takes gender, race, and age into consideration, it is easier to grasp the levels of social inequality in the country. During the pandemic, the people who took the biggest hit in several different aspects – economically, socially, and in terms of health – were the women, the Black and indigenous populations, as well as the elderly who had the higher risk of hospitalisation and death due to their age.

This chapter aims to analyse through a critical perspective the struggle for the guarantee of rights and reduction of social inequalities in Rio de Janeiro's favelas. It takes as a starting point the complex situations that emerged with the pandemic, emphasising that even in the face of government techno-politics that drive up the death rates of poor people, Black people, and slum dwellers, territorial insurgencies indicate other paths for the construction of a dignified life and access to basic rights. These paths are guided by practices of solidarity, territorial political organisation, and the construction of specific public policies to deal with the effects of the virus, taking into consideration the particularities and distinct realities across the territory.

In this chapter, we refer to the concept of "territory" developed by Milton Santos (2001), a Brazilian geographer. Santos (2001) emphasises that territory should not be understood only as a material space, but also as the relations of force established in that space. The territory is simultaneously material and social, it is not a static form, it is a dynamic, living, and interacting space. As Santos (2001) states:

> "Territory is not just the result of the superposition of a set of natural systems and a set of systems of things created by man [sic]. The territory is the ground plus the population, that is, an identity, the fact and the feeling of belonging to what belongs to us. The territory is the basis of work, residence, and the material and spiritual exchanges and of life, which it influences" (p. 47).

In this scenario, the markers of territorial difference emerge as a factor that can hinder or leverage the resources for carrying out the work of community articulation. From this perspective, we analysed the actions to fight the coronavirus in a slum in Rio de Janeiro called Fumacê. We conducted qualitative interviews with Rogéria Xavier, a community organiser. Rogéria is a Black woman who lives in Fumacê, has over 20 years of experience in the community and has promoted effective actions to fight and prevent the consequences of the pandemic since its beginning. The experiences of articulation and community organisation in the slums led by local groups and supporting institutions have guaranteed the distribution of food and personal hygiene items, the sanitation of alleys and alleyways, the distribution of information about the virus to the population and political coordination for disputes in defence of life in the slums, in the face of genocidal processes carried out by the Federal Government.

Who is Rogéria?

Rogéria Xavier is 46 years old and lives in Rio de Janeiro, born and raised in the territory of Fumacê. Rogéria represents the strength of Black women who support families (hers and other people's). She is a mother, grandmother, nurse, and community organiser, who was part of the local "Homeowners" association' for six years. Due to her previous work in the community, mostly in local schools, she started a job over nine years ago as an "agent of civic values" in the field of social responsibility at a private company.

To understand the strength of Rogéria's representativity, it is necessary to adopt an intersectional lens and an understanding of social markers of difference (Piscitelli, 2008, Ferreira, 2014; Zamboni, 2014). Gender is a social marker of difference just like race/ethnicity, social class, age, sexual orientation, territory, among others. Such markers arrange ways of understanding the world, social relations, and power structures. They influence the subject's perception of themselves. Labels are generally dichotomous and contribute to social ranking and the production of inequalities based on the denial or discrimination of the other. The ways in which people exist and act in the world are produced and legitimised through the hegemonic functioning of these markers, and those who disassociate from these established patterns are likely to become excluded and/or criminalised.

These different categories intersect and their permutations influence different areas, such as: the quality of access to basic rights guaranteed in the federal constitution; the perception and exercise of citizenship; and the fight for dignified living conditions. When we consider Rogéria's trajectory, we see her effort to promote the access of favela residents to their rights and improvements in the favela where they live. From the beginning of the pandemic, Rogéria focused on actions to mitigate and combat detrimental health, social and economic effects on her territory. Like many Brazilians, she and her family suffered from the consequences of Covid-19. She reported the death of her 46-year-old brother and the mental illness of family members, *"depression came into my house, and I was strong, but my mother wasn't, she still hasn't recovered"*.

In Brazil, the first confirmed death from Covid-19 happened in Rio de Janeiro: a 63-year-old Black woman called Cleonice Golçalves who worked as a housemaid and suffered from comorbidities like diabetes and hypertension (Cruz, 2021). She worked in the Leblon neighbourhood, in the South Zone of the city, where property prices are among the most expensive in the country. Her employer had recently returned from Italy infected with the virus. Cleonice Gonçalves' skin colour was only recently confirmed. Cleonice was one of the Black women who were victims of Covid-19 and were omitted and made invisible (Brandão, 2021).

In Brazil and around the world, during the pandemic, Black women were at even greater social vulnerability (Iraci et al., 2018; UNFPA, 2020). The pandemic amplified the inequalities generated by the current dominant economic model. If women and men were equally represented in the job market, 112 million women would no longer be at risk of losing their income or work. In Brazil, Black people are 40% more likely to die from Covid-19 than White people (Werneck et al., 2021).

Black women are also at the centre of many social assistance policies, including cash transfer programs. During the pandemic, this remained the case in several food collection campaigns. As an example, we highlight the *Mães de Favela* ("Mothers from the Slums") campaign, proposed in 2020 by the *Central Única de Favelas* (CUFA), based on research conducted by the *Locomotiva* Institute and *Data Favela* (institutions dedicated to study favelas and run census-like research with their inhabitants). This research pointed out that Brazil's favelas have 5.2 million mothers and projected that more than 70% of them would be without income during lockdown periods. Research published by the BBC News Brazil (Guimarães, 2020), emphasised the social role and vulnerability of women living in favelas in supporting and caring for their children and elders from an intersectional perspective:

"The most fragile in society are the slum dwellers. The most fragile among the slum dwellers are the women. And the most fragile among women are mothers. Why? Because they take care of their children, they often work in informal jobs, sewing, doing nails, and they still provide care for the old. Because all the old people, 90% of the elderly in the slums, are cared for by women: either daughters or daughters-in-law"

(Guimarães, 2020).

During the pandemic, Rogéria was the main carer and income source for her entire family, while she simultaneously developed important community actions as she acknowledged the effects of the pandemic in her territory. Ethnographic research conducted with popular leaders of the Health Promotion Network (RCS) of the metropolitan area of Rio de Janeiro highlighted the power of agency, organisation, and emancipation of women from socially excluded segments, mainly poor and Black, aged between 30 and 59 years old (Mello e Souza et al., 2018). Among the engaged leaders, 52% had been activists for 6 to 15 years (Mello e Souza et al., 2018). Black women face situations of multiple vulnerabilities, and they resist these situations, constructing a position of struggle and social transformation. Rogéria stated:

"I consider myself a community organiser. Because leadership is often about being present in [a community] that is ready [for social change] and not [yet] engaged [in it]. For example: community services like water and sewage, and an articulation that go beyond [those services], it's like creating bridges between the community and the health sector, the education sector … it's talking directly to the masses and instilling an idea of change within the social area, it's articulating [people and organisations] in the territory".

When Rogéria describes the community work done in Fumacê, she uses powerful verbs such as build, engage, change, and articulate. Here, "territory" is an important category of analysis, since it is in the territory that Rogéria develops her actions, establishes her relationships, and is affected both by experiences of difficulties and violations of rights, as well as by movements of recognition from the residents. *"Because it is gratifying to do this, to look and see that a young person, a housewife went there, thought about changing her life, studying and becoming an entrepreneur because she listened to me, it is priceless"*. The favela territory is a place of multiple connections and is also configured as an existential territory.

Most of the favelas arose due to the brutal imposition of inequality on workers, limiting their access to fundamental rights such as the right to housing (Valle et al., 2015). Throughout the history of the slums, their residents have constantly pressured public authorities to demand improvements. They have often received negligence and violence as a response, for example with the demolition of houses, in alleged public safety projects, and the breakdown of democratic dialogues with the population. Since the early 20th century, the Brazilian public authorities perceive the slum as a problem to be extinguished or at least controlled in the context of its population growth (Melicio et al., 2012).

Thus, the logic of "we for us" prevails in many of these territories, not as a dead phrase, but as a daily practice of invention of a world where life is possible. This echoes a philosophy of existence that is guided by sharing, the strengthening of the collective, the principles of "ubuntu". Ubuntu is an African philosophy that proposes an ethos of solidarity and interdependence with others:

> "Ubuntu situates individuals within a web of relationships that is born of identifying with others and acting in solidarity. It is by sharing a way of life with others that individuals 'come into existence'. We exist because our social connections remain strong, extending beyond family to embrace our clan, village and entire community"
>
> (Seifu Estifanos et al., 2020, p.1).

In this sense, the concept and phenomenon of territory is essential in this discussion. Being a slum dweller may mean experiencing discrimination and a violation of one's rights. But living in the slum also implies experiencing other forms of sociability, coexistence with diversity, multiple crossings that generate power, resistance, and the possibility of social change. Rogéria states that:

> "*The actors arise from the needs of the place. Here [working] with me I have a young man, Reginaldo, who provides sports practice to more than 100 children, he pays for it out of his own pocket. I have another resident named Bruno Black who through cultural activities is gradually changing the minds of the local people and talking about Fumacê all over Brazil*".

The name of the favela, Fumacê, which means "smoke" or "fog", came from the fact that in previous decades many residents did not have gas stoves, so they used stoves that emitted so much smoke that they could be seen from far away (José, 2017). The territory was for a long time considered one of the most violent in the entire state of Rio de Janeiro. In 2012, it received a Police Pacifying Unit (UPP), which made the number of social projects increase in the place. After the deactivation of the local UPP, conflicts between rival criminal gangs for the control of drug dealing in the region intensified, along with a decrease in projects taking place in the territory.

In the pandemic, many existing projects stopped as a result of the lockdown, as did some social projects, and many merchants closed the doors of their small businesses. Favelas and poorer areas have in entrepreneurship (by desire, and mostly by necessity) one of the main sources of economic development. Rogéria pointed out that with the closing of small businesses, unemployment has grown in the area, "*I saw the fearful expression of those who had nothing and no one to ask for help*".

The city of Rio de Janeiro has the largest number of people living in slums in the whole country, representing 22.03% of the population. A comparison of the 2010 Census with the 2000 Census reveals that this population increased by 27.5%. Since the beginning of the pandemic, legislative initiatives at all government levels have been proposed to contain the spread of the virus in the slums. Many of these initiatives were created in dialogue with social movements and universities, aiming to propose emergency care plans for these vulnerable places. They were based in the understanding that, in the face of the pandemic, the state should take responsibility for ensuring the minimum for a dignified life during lockdown periods. These measures included broad issues such as access to water, food, and minimum income, as well as the safety of the residents, with the prohibition of police operations in the slums while the pandemic was ongoing.

Faced with the consequences of the pandemic in the territory of Fumacê, Rogéria focused on the strategy of articulating and strengthening the network of people, activists, and organisations, carrying out actions, mainly, with local residents and groups from the private sector. Rogéria joined the *União Rio* (Union Rio) Movement and the *Rio Contra Corona* (Rio Against Coronavirus) projects, which were important achievements. Based on these partnerships, she was able to develop important actions in the territory. The actions were mainly on three fronts: i) means of prevention; ii) reduction of food insecurity; and iii) reliable information.

i   Aiming to help with access to the means of prevention and contamination reduction and with donations from partner companies, Rogéria distributed masks, more than two thousand units of alcohol gel, and hygiene and cleaning products.

ii   With the closing of shops, reduced work possibilities, especially for the self-employed and delay in the payment of emergency aid, many families entered a situation of food insecurity. In this scenario, ensuring the donations of basic food parcels was important work, which helped more than 8,000 families. Referring to government and the public services, Rogéria stated that *"nobody came to do anything, no one came to do any work"*.

iii   In collaboration with private companies, Rogéria has conducted educational prevention actions. She ensured access to printed educational materials and has distributed leaflets about prevention actions such as hand washing and social distancing. She has been talking to young people about the risk of sharing cigarettes. One of the measures taken by Rogéria was a partnership with a *Clínica da Família*, a public health unit that is focused on primary health care for the poorer population and had an important role in the vaccination campaign across the territory. Therefore, Rogeria, with all her community engagement power, reinforced the importance of immunisation and the use of face masks.

As pointed out by Mello e Souza et al. (2018), since they live in the targeted territory, leaders, and/or community organisers act simultaneously as agents and public of their actions. The demands and aches of the residents often intersect with their own. Through social connection and daily interaction, individual and collective bonds are sewed and strengthened. The feeling of community is formed through inhabiting the same territory. Fuelled by the government's carelessness, the effects of the pandemic and the need for action, resilience, power of coordination, and social activism emerge as vital forces in the face of the inequalities experienced.

Final Thoughts

The pandemic turned its spotlight on Brazilian social issues, exposing and intensifying them, such as the amount of people experiencing food insecurity, the increase in unemployment and (at the time of writing) the death of 652,000 Brazilians because of the pandemic and severe social inequality. These processes showed the cruel effects of a government that uses denial and negligence in a moment of crisis and health emergency.

Nonetheless, the pandemic shone a light on the work of articulation and social coordination that has been undertaken by many different people, mainly the inhabitants of the favelas and outskirts of the city. Many are the Carioca (from the city of Rio) and Brazilian Rogérias that have a history of community work. The social work and growth of the third sector and civil society organisation in Brazil gained strength with the 1988 Constitution, but in the favelas and poorer areas these movements of solidarity and political pressure have always been present.

It is worth questioning who is *centro* (the city centre or the "centre" of the city) and who is in the "periphery" (the rundown areas far away from the city centre) in terms of citizenship and sense of community. The truths and subjectivities produced about these territories are configured as an arena of dispute, in a movement of tension and conformity between what is established and what will establish new possibilities of understanding the world. This dispute includes movements that focus on challenging classist, sexist, and racist stereotypes related to subordination, inability, and discredit concerning the status of citizen.

Ogien (2018) argues that the periphery perspective may be seen as a claim for democracy. Regarding the distinctions between centre and periphery, the geographer Jailson de Souza e Silva (2012), in his open letter to the Brazilian writer Zuenir Ventura criticizing the concept of the broken city, points out that citizenship is not a point of arrival, but rather a starting point and a permanent construction. He claims that it might be more adequate to speak of a "broken State", dominated by the interests of specific social groups, and not fulfilling its supposed "universal role". He argues that slum and suburban dwellers have always had to move around the city in search of their basic rights, just as it happened again during the pandemic, and pressure the government to fulfil its obligations. What is needed is the awareness of the government and the market about the need for access to fundamental rights, but, as Silva (2012) emphasises, "the poor have always been aware of this and have sought, by legitimate or illegitimate means, to guarantee these rights" (p. 21).

Deleuze (2010, p. 222) stated that "Believing in the world is what we lack the most; we have completely lost the world, we have been dispossessed of it". Individuals can or cannot become subjects of their utterances and practices, can or cannot confront meaninglessness. What can we strive for? Proposing new experiences of space-time, even on reduced surfaces or volumes, considering the effects of the encounters, always unknown beforehand, are somehow still micropolitical propositions: something like attempting to recover the world.

Resistance practices open space for difference as they share and inquire ways of existence. From their own mechanisms – most of the time inapprehensible – one can enable the development of new possibilities of life. It is important to resignify social rights through other perspectives, understanding them also as distinct ways of feeling, existing, thinking, and being in the world.

References

Brandão, F. (2021, november 11). *Pesquisadores cobram dados sobre mulheres negras vítimas de Covid-19*. Agência Câmara de Notícias. https://www.camara.leg.br/noticias/709315-pesquisadores-cobram-dados-sobre-mulheres-negras-vitimas-de-covid-19/

Cruz, P.S.G. (2021, june 15) *De Marielle Franco a Cleonice Gonçalves e Miguel: a interseccionalidade como ferramenta analítica na elaboração* de políticas públicas efetivas. FE PUBLICA. https://www.fe.unicamp.br/fe-publica/publicacoes/de-marielle-franco-a-cleonice-goncalves-e-miguel-a-interseccionalidade-0

Deleuze, G., & Guattari, F. (2010). *A máquina capitalista civilizada. O anti-Édipo: capitalismo e esquizofrenia*. São Paulo: Ed. 34, 295–317.

Ferreira, G.G. (2014). Interseccionalidades e marcadores sociais da diferença na experiência de travestis privadas de liberdade. *Anais do II Seminário Regional Políticas Públicas*. Porto Alegre: EdUFRGS. https://editora.pucrs.br/edipucrs/anais/serpinf/2014/assets/23.pdf

Galindo, M. (2020). *Desobediencia, por tu culpa voy a sobrevivir. Sopa de Wuhan*. Buenos Aires: Aspo Editorial, 119–128.

Guimarães, L. (2020, april 2). *Coronavírus: 92% das mães nas favelas dizem que faltará comida após um mês de isolamento, aponta pesquisa*. BBC News Brasil. https://www.bbc.com/portuguese/brasil-52131989

Iraci, N. et al. (2018). A Situação dos Direitos Humanos das Mulheres Negras no Brasil - Violências e Violações. In: *Dossiê Geledés*. Instituto da Mulher Negra e Criola. Organização de Mulheres Negras. 2017. https://www.geledes.org.br/dossie-situacao-direitos-humanos-mulheres-negras-brasil-violencias-violacoes/?gclid=CjwKCAjwquWVBhBrEiwAt1Kmwt_Ly6KKzp91UlP2wmz3nuucumkeEuX20cIlnXgQofejGh4zuMJfvhoCJLQQAvD_BwE

José, F. (2017, july 6). *Afinal, por que Fumacê?*. Voz das Comunidades. https://www.vozdascomunidades.com.br/geral/afinal-por-que-fumace/

Melicio, T.B.L., Geraldini, J.R., & Bicalho, P.P.G. (2012). *Biopoder e UPPs: alteridade na experiência do policiamento permanente em comunidades cariocas*. Fractal: Revista de Psicologia, *24*(3), 599–622. https://www.scielo.br/j/fractal/a/9yQ7cfB6tGxHNCnRLVgdxXQ/abstract/?lang=pt

Mbembé, J.A., & Meintjes, L. (2003). Necropolitics. *Public culture*, *15*(1), 11–40. https://muse.jhu.edu/article/39984/pdf

Mello e Souza, C. et al. (2018). Movimentos populares e motivações de lideranças comunitárias: agência, reconhecimento e transformação de si e do coletivo. In Maciel, T.B. & Mello e Souza, C. (Org). *Inovação e trajetos: comunidade, desenvolvimento e sustentabilidade.* Curitiba: Appris, 23–44. ISBN 9788547325145.

Ogien, A. (2018). Uma concepção expandida de Periferia. *Periferias, 1*(2). https://revistaperiferias.org/

OXFAM Brasil (2021). *O vírus da desigualdade 2021.* https://materiais.oxfam.org.br/o-virus-da-desigualdade

Piscitelli, A. (2008). Interseccionalidades, categorias de articulação e experiências de migrantes brasileiras. *Sociedade e Cultura, 11*(2), 263–274. 10.5216/sec.v11i2.5247

Santos, M. (2001). *Por uma outra globalização*: do pensamento único à consciência universal. Rio de Janeiro: Record. ISBN:6555871865

Seifu Estifanos, A., Alemu, G., Negussie, S. et al. (2020). 'I exist because of we': shielding as a communal ethic of maintaining social bonds during the COVID-19 response in Ethiopia. *BMJ Global Health, 5*, e003204. 10.1136/ bmjgh-2020-003204

Silva, J.S. (2012) *O novo carioca.* Rio de Janeiro: Mórula Editorial. ISBN: 6559210405

UNFPA - United Nations Fund for Population Activities (2020). *State of World Population 2020: Against my will - Defying the practices that harm women and girls and undermine equality.* https://www.unfpa.org/sites/default/files/pub-pdf/UNFPA_PUB_2020_EN_State_of_World_Population.pdf

Valle, L.F., Cunha, T.C., & Bicalho, P.P.G. (2015). Les inventions clinico-politiques dans l'intervention de la psychologie dans la favela. *Bulletin de Psychologie, 68*(2), 125–132. 10.3917/bupsy.536.0125

Werneck, G.L., Bahia, L., Moreira, J.P.L., & Scheffer, M. (2021). Mortes evitáveis por Covid-19 no Brasil. *Movimento Alerta.* https://www.oxfam.org.br/especiais/mortes-evitaveis-por-covid-19-no-brasil/

Zamboni, M. (2014). Marcadores Sociais da Diferença. *Sociologia: grandes temas do conhecimento, 1*, 14–18. https://edisciplinas.usp.br/mod/resource/view.php?id=3040037&forceview=1

4 Volunteering Motivation to Combat Covid-19: Evidence from Community Responses in China

Susan Schwarz, Gary Schwarz, and Qing Miao

Introduction

The Covid-19 pandemic has negatively impacted the lives of billions of people around the world, increasing mortality rates, inequality, and isolation while restricting access for many to basic education and human services. During such widespread public crisis, community response activities require rapid, broad coordination among a range of actors, including government, non-profit organisations (NPOs), and individual citizens (Comfort et al., 2001; Feduzi et al., 2022; Wu et al., 2021). In addition, the demands of Covid-19 have threatened the financial viability of NPOs striving to alleviate the consequences of the pandemic for the most vulnerable populations, thereby exacerbating the problems (Maher et al., 2020). Under such crisis conditions, NPOs rely more than ever on citizen volunteers who devote their own time and efforts to support others in their communities (Rotolo & Berg, 2011).

But how can NPOs mobilise and engage volunteers effectively and productively? What motivations drive volunteers – particularly experienced volunteers who can provide high-quality professionalised services to fill critical gaps created by Covid? What factors influence participation in community response? In this chapter, we focus at the micro level on volunteering frequency and intensity, motivation, including efficacy and social ties, the role of digital technology, and the professionalisation of volunteering in the context of East Asia during the pandemic's first wave.

Following the initial outbreak of Covid-19 in central China, the virus spread swiftly as the country began its most important annual holiday, the Spring Festival (Zhang et al., 2020). Volunteerism in response to the pandemic began slowly and then gained rapid momentum, facilitated by numerous factors. This study examines factors driving this mobilisation, including the role of NPOs and local volunteers working to protect public health in response to the Covid-19 outbreak. We draw on volunteer motivation and emergency management literature to understand how such efforts can be rallied to support community services while also laying the groundwork for future research in this domain.

Our research makes several contributions at the conceptual and practical levels. Our exploration of volunteer motivation during the pandemic contributes

DOI: 10.4324/9781003301905-5

to understanding efficacy, salience, and social factors as drivers of engagement. The role of professionalised volunteers provides insights into the application of human capital to support public services during crisis events. On a practical level, our research can help NPOs combatting pandemics – and other major crises around the world – improve their partnerships with individual volunteers through evidence-based practices. Such practices can help improve the standard of living of those affected by the pandemic and maintain or enhance the quality of services during emergencies. Finally, we demonstrate the value of mobile technology and social media to mobilise and engage with volunteers, especially during events that require social distancing and remote communication.

The rest of this chapter is structured as follows: Section 2 provides a brief background on volunteerism and the Chinese context, and a glimpse of the literature related to volunteer engagement and motivation. In Section 3, we describe the methods used to collect quantitative and qualitative data from Covid-19 volunteers and organisations in China. Section 4 presents the findings, relating them to research and practice. Finally, in Section 5, we conclude by discussing the implications of our findings and providing re-commendations on how to further explore these topics going forward.

Conceptual Background and Context

In a broad-based definition, Wilson (2012) views volunteering work as ac-tivities in which unpaid time and assistance are freely given to benefit other people, causes, groups, or organisations. Volunteerism is considered valuable for providing services, building civic morale and responsibility, and enhancing the community (Hustinx et al., 2012). Governments often promote vo-lunteering as a matter of policy to help provide needed support and benefits to communities (Stukas et al., 2016). Volunteer efforts by citizens, in co-ordination with government, can strengthen community and regional resi-lience during major emergencies by providing a kind of flexible "surge capacity" that closes emergency gaps in times of extreme demand (McLennan et al., 2016). NPOs can help public agencies extend skill sets by deploying knowledgeable volunteers and offering empathetic client contact within the community (Nesbit et al., 2018), especially during crises.

Volunteering has been rising in China in the past three decades due to the government's efforts to encourage citizen participation to gain legitimacy and establish a state-endorsed civil society (Hustinx et al., 2012; Wu et al., 2018). Volunteering gained momentum in China in the aftermath of the Sichuan earthquake, the Beijing Olympics, and the Shanghai World Expo, which de-monstrated that volunteers can be deployed successfully for disaster relief and important events (Hu et al., 2016; Wang & Wu, 2014). Volunteer schemes were created to realise the benefit of volunteerism, with voluntary service organisa-tions frequently serving as implementors of both policy and services (Hu, 2021). Motivating citizens to serve as volunteers is thus considered a task of national importance, particularly during a pandemic.

In the Chinese context, volunteerism exhibits features of both top-down state direction and bottom-up local orchestration (Wu et al., 2018). Government volunteering schemes such as the Guidance on Building Social Service Volunteer Teams in China: 2013–2020 and the State Council's 2017 Volunteer Service Ordinance have been enacted to increase individual volunteer participation at the regional and community levels (Hu, 2021). In recent years, voluntary participation has also been fostered by social media innovations, including the introduction of a popular volunteering digital app, ZhiYuanHui ("Volunteering Together"). The two-sided mobile platform allows individual volunteers to locate nearby service opportunities while helping NPOs find volunteers. The app was released for free public use in 2015 by the high-tech firm ZhongQingYixin, located in Hangzhou, and became the most widely used voluntary social media app in China. By 2020, just prior to Covid's first wave, the number of registered users had reached 78 million individuals and 400,000 NPOs across China.

Motivating Volunteers

Motivating volunteers has long been considered a crucial task for NPOs globally as they seek to mobilise volunteers (Harrison, 1995). A clear understanding of volunteer motivation can help organisations better target recruitment and retention efforts, ensuring effective deployment (Stukas et al., 2016). Empirical work finds that external social influences, including subjective norms and internal moral obligations, are strong determinants of volunteer motivation (Harrison, 1995), with "other" rather than "self" oriented values linked to volunteer commitment (Stukas et al., 2016). An empirical study across 27 Chinese cities found the strongest predictor of volunteerism was norms of generalised reciprocity, or belief in doing good in the community (Wu et al., 2018). Similarly, scholars find that important factors in voluntary activity include a sense of responsibility and empathy for others (Wilhelm & Bekkers, 2010) and communally oriented values (Finkelstein, 2010).

Motivation is also linked with the salience of the activities because citizens' attention must first be attracted for them to respond to an important issue (McDonald, 2009). For instance, proximity to a problem or the influence of social ties may serve to capture peoples' attention (Rotolo & Berg, 2011). Major crises provide this combination of urgency and relevance to make citizen engagement salient (Gazley & Brudney, 2005). Motivation is also linked to a sense of self-efficacy in terms of individuals perceiving they possess the ability to make a difference or have an impact (Einolf, 2008; Schwarz et al., 2021).

Professionalisation of Volunteers

The deployment of professionalised, experienced "veteran" volunteers can help extend service delivery in times of urgency, apply needed skills, and provide direct client service "on the ground" in local areas (Gazley & Brudney, 2005; Van Eijk & Steen, 2014). For instance, participation may be driven (or hampered) by volunteers' ability to contribute skilled resources such as knowledge and experience (Sundeen et al., 2007). Professional experience, especially in previous crisis management, is a key element in developing adaptive capacity at both the individual and organisational levels (Comfort et al., 2001). On a macro level, effective deployment of this experience helps preserve the gains of development and living standards, which have been compromised in many countries because of pandemic-induced economic losses.

Methods

To explore the above topics, we collected our data in Zhejiang Province. Adjacent to Shanghai, this area of eastern China offered an important context for our study. Geographically, the province is just one-third of the size of Italy, but its population is nearly the same – in the range of 60 million people. In 2020, Zhejiang faced high risks from Covid-19 because of its dense and mobile population and its status as an active entrepreneurial, digital, and manufacturing hub generating frequent interaction.

The data for our study were gathered from three sources. First, we analysed usage data from 85,699 people who volunteered between 21 January and 22 February 2020, at the very outset of the Covid-19 pandemic. Data were obtained from the ZhiYuanHui volunteering digital app launched in 2015 by ZhongQingYixin company, which provides volunteer registration and service recording in addition to basic volunteer insurance and a social media platform to share stories and photos.

Second, to understand the background, drivers, and behaviour of dedicated volunteers, we conducted an online survey with 1,889 volunteers who had volunteered before the pandemic and continued to do so during the crisis. These volunteers were registered on the digital volunteering app ZhiYuanHui between 2015 and early 2020. We randomly targeted 5,000 active volunteers using a pop-up survey, with 37.78% of these individuals responding during the first quarter of 2020.

Finally, we conducted 14 semi-structured one-to-one interviews with non-profit managers coordinating voluntary activities in Zhejiang Province during the pandemic. They also worked as volunteers themselves and thus had significant experience within the region and local communities. Our sample included a geographically diverse group of non-profit managers leading relief efforts in each of the province's 11 prefecture-level cities. We selected the largest local NPO in these cities and invited the director of each organisation for an interview. We conducted additional interviews with another NPO director from the cities most severely affected by Covid-19 (Wenzhou, Taizhou, and the capital Hangzhou). Each interview lasted approximately half an hour.

Results: "We Worked with One Heart"

Our findings across the three data sources revealed numerous details and nuances regarding volunteer activity, characteristics of the volunteers, and motivational factors in the pandemic's early stages. Among the Zhejiang volunteers, Covid-19 service work included a broad range of practical tasks and responsibilities. These included disseminating supplies such as personal protective equipment, food, drinks, and pharmaceuticals to frontline staff in medical and security settings; providing support, such as transportation and food distribution, to vulnerable populations and families; conducting logistical and technical tasks to back up health care workers and pandemic centres; and disseminating information and training on public health practices via telephone hotlines and Internet platforms, typically within the local community.

Overall Volunteer Trend

Statistics on the overall volunteering rate from the mobile app provide a snapshot of the emerging crisis. While volunteerism was slightly dampened at first because of the Spring Festival holiday, participation grew rapidly as the pandemic took hold in eastern China. Notably, on 21 January, volunteer numbers were extremely low as residents prepared for the Lunar New Year on 25 January (Zhang et al., 2020). Soon afterwards, however, volunteer activity began to rise, keeping pace with the growing infection rate (see Figure 4.1).

Volunteering Frequency and Intensity

Based on the digital app for all ZhiYuanHui volunteers, average service hours grew each day, from 5.2 hours on 21 January to 6.9 hours on 22 February (see Figure 4.2). Likewise, the number of projects self-allocated by volunteers rose from 1.23 to 1.43 daily. Meanwhile, the volunteering frequency, or average

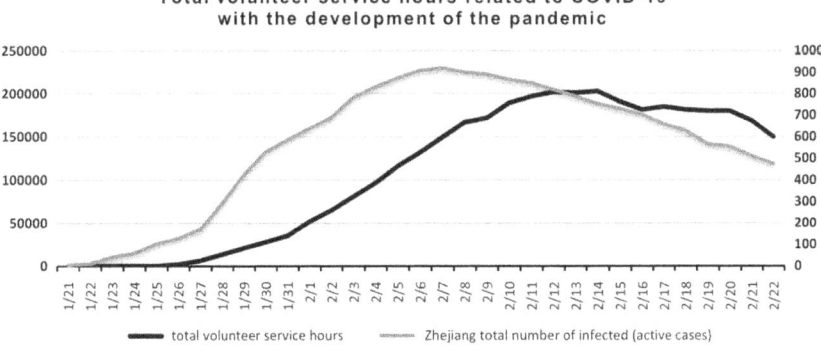

Figure 4.1 Covid-19 related volunteer service hours and pandemic progression (January–February 2020).

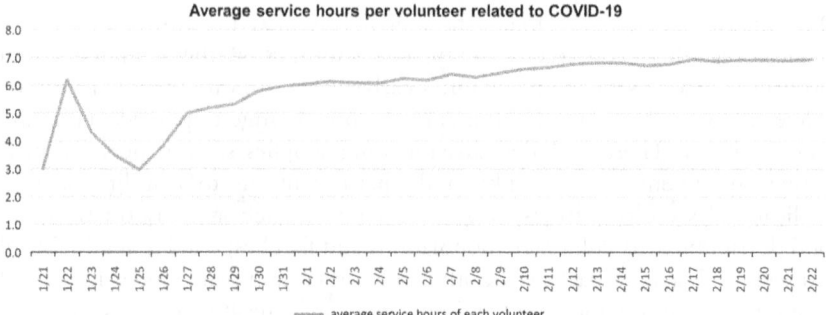

Figure 4.2 Covid-19 related average volunteer service hours per day (January–February 2020).

number of shifts per week, was 4.16, with nearly one-third (32.6%) volunteering seven times per week – an impressive level of commitment we designated as "super-hero" volunteering. In addition, nearly 40% (38.9%) reported volunteering for seven or more hours per shift, with more than 70% volunteering for at least 5 hours per shift. About 10% of the volunteers worked nightshifts.

Notably, in response to the urgent crisis beginning in late January, experienced volunteers already active on the app shifted over from previous causes, such as special education or ecological concerns, to focus on virus relief efforts. Among these regular volunteers, nearly 70% stated that they volunteered more frequently than before the pandemic.

Volunteer Motivation and Engagement

The app and survey data both indicated motivations that appeared to drive the volunteers: immediacy and salience, self-efficacy, social ties, and the availability of professional skills that could be deployed for volunteering tasks. These were further reflected in comments from the NPO leaders in the interviews.

Immediacy and Salience

The switching-over of existing volunteers towards Covid-19 and away from previous causes suggests immediacy and salience of a cause as a strong motivator (Beyerlein & Sikkink, 2008). The urgency and uniqueness of the crisis were noted by one non-profit manager: "As soon as the outbreak in January started, we considered it was definitely different from the ordinary snowstorm or earthquake" (Interview 10). In response to unfolding events, a second NPO leader commented: "Because we are aware of the seriousness of the epidemic, we as volunteer organisations should participate as much as possible. At the beginning, publicity was carried out on the first and second day of the (Lunar) New Year to make more people realise the severity of the epidemic and call for people to participate" (Interview 6). Another observed: "When our country got caught off-guard in a crisis, we were ready to help out. When they're in need, we will be out there" (Interview 5). No tangible compensation was expected. One NPO leader commented: "There is no subsidy from the government, and there will be a box of instant noodles if you are on duty at night" (Interview 2).

Self-Efficacy, Community, and Social Ties

The strongest motivation reported by Covid-19 volunteers was confidence in their ability to make a difference, or efficacy. The survey results revealed that 96% of the 1,889 respondents cited their main motivation as efficacy: "I believe my participation can do something good for controlling the epidemic". Volunteers' desire and belief in their ability to make a difference was a key driver of subsequent volunteer engagement. Those individuals who were motivated to "do something good" to address the pandemic volunteered more than those driven by other motivations (e.g., career or personal benefit, social interaction with friends, or getting out of the house). In the survey, a statistically significant difference was seen between volunteers with different motivations in terms of greater volunteering frequency (times per week) $[F(4/1884) = 3.82, p = .004]$ and intensity (hours per shift) $[F(4/1884) = 2.43, p = .046]$. Likewise, interview comments reflected interest and belief in making a difference. For example, "In the current epidemic, medical personnel are fighting on the front line, and many ordinary people in the rear are silently devoting their strength. As ordinary people, we are happy and proud to be able to participate in such voluntary work, and hope that the epidemic will disappear as soon as possible" [Interview 4].

Closely linked to this desire for impact, volunteers were also motivated by a sense of duty and responsibility for community service and contributing to the amelioration of the crisis. One manager commented: "People think it is worthwhile to make a contribution to their community or village as a volunteer. Our motives are unpaid and selfless. Everyone was very enthusiastic" (Interview 3). Another observed, "Responding to the need of the community, we help to meet it ... Ordinary people are willing to make a personal contribution to the society" (Interview 9).

Close ties among personal networks may also inspire volunteer action (Wu et al., 2018), with nearly 70% of survey respondents reporting that relatives were also volunteering. This result is consistent with previous findings that "bonding" social networks increase the likelihood of volunteering (Wilson, 2012). Those with relatives also volunteering in Zhejiang had significantly greater volunteering frequency $[F(1/1887) = 34.83, p < .001]$ and volunteering intensity $[F(1/1887) = 25.82, p < .001]$, suggesting that close ties play an important role in volunteer engagement. Indeed, among the leaders interviewed, several commented on connections among existing and new volunteers, for instance, noting, "We are also recruiting volunteers from our own group of friends" [Interview 8].

Bringing together these findings on self-efficacy, community, and social ties suggests insights into the individual–society relationship in this context. While much of the Zhejiang volunteering was inspired if not initiated, at least in-directly, at the behest of state organisations, volunteer turnout involved significant bottom-up as well as top-down efforts. The use of the digital app fostered decentralisation, with volunteers engaging "at will" and working for a range of different NPOs. Deployment was largely at the local level through grassroots organisations, for instance with municipal and regional governments requesting their support. In some cases, non-profits led the way, taking action before the crisis was fully acknowledged or a widespread plan formulated. One local leader commented, "We acted first. We took the initiative to contact the government. When the epidemic was gradually exposed, they began to look for us actively. Generally speaking, we walked in front of the government" (Interview 10).

In addition, broader plans emerging at the township or county level were often implemented through grassroots outreach. For instance, Interviewee 10, director of an emergency NPO in Taizhou, noted eclectic efforts to mobilise the work of diverse volunteers. Experienced middle-aged volunteers oversaw hands-on relief efforts in the field, at times in concert with small business owners who had time and expertise (e.g., for distribution of materials). Meanwhile, elderly people leveraged community and government contacts from the safety of home, while students and younger people with Internet skills engaged in collecting data and disseminating digital information. From a collective perspective, we would describe the overall phenomenon as "in-spired top-down and implemented bottom-up".

Professional Skills

Occupational background, education, and experience were notable factors among the Covid-19 volunteers. In terms of professional life, the volunteers came from a broad range of occupational sectors, including public institutes, private companies, students, state-owned firms, and NPO/non-governmental organisations (NGOs) (see Table 4.1).

Occupational speciality influenced volunteering **engagement**, with NPO/NGO employees volunteering the most (in addition to their paid employment within the sector) and students volunteering the least, in terms of both frequency [$F(11/1877) = 12.09$, $p < .001$] and intensity [$F(1/1887) = 34.83$, $p < .001$]. In addition, more than half (57.5%) of the volunteers had completed higher education at the junior college, undergraduate, or postgraduate levels, with another 23% holding senior middle or specialised secondary (upper secondary) diplomas, bringing this knowledge to their volunteer service (see Table 4.2).

Table 4.1 Occupation of volunteers

Volunteer Occupation (Sector)	Subtotal	Proportion
Public institutes (education, science, culture, health)	330	17.47%
Freelance	316	16.73%
Private companies	270	14.27%
Students	188	9.96%
State-owned companies	170	8.98%
Retired	158	8.36%
NPO/NGO	105	5.54%
Others	100	5.29%
Public servants	98	5.17%
Entrepreneurs	98	5.17%
Not working currently	39	2.09%
Foreign companies	19	0.98%
Total	1889	

Table 4.2 Education level of volunteers

Education Level Completed	Subtotal	Proportion
Primary school	32	1.72%
Junior middle school	337	17.84%
Senior middle school	300	15.87%
Secondary specialised school	135	7.13%
Junior college	469	24.85%
Undergraduate	579	30.63%
Postgraduate	37	1.97%
Total	1889	

Those individuals with more volunteering background prior to the pandemic tended to contribute significantly more during the crisis – those who had been registered longer on the ZhiYuanHui app (i.e., 2015–2020) were seen to volunteer more frequently each week [$F(5/2262) = 15.92$, $p < .001$] and for longer stints [$F(5/2262) = 16.97$, $p < .001$].

Comments from NPO leaders indicated they value these long-term volunteers who contribute professional skills, for instance, gained through paid employment or previous volunteering. One NPO leader commented, "Volunteering now is not the same as it used to be. Now, volunteering must have a speciality or professionalism ... The volunteers here are more professional; they all have strong skills" (Interview 10). Others noted, "Most members of our team are long-term volunteers" (Interview 6) and "The participation of professional volunteers gives us more confidence" (Interview 12). Reflecting the theme of professionalisation, a large welfare service organisation in southeast Zhejiang organised online training for 500 community groups on "how to achieve professional and orderly volunteer service during the epidemic" (Interview 11).

Table 4.3 Exemplary quotes from non-profit leaders

Key Theme	Exemplary Quotes
Salience and Relevance of Crisis	When our country got caught off-guard in a crisis, we're ready to help out. When they're in need, we will be out there. [Int 5]
	Because we are aware of the seriousness of the epidemic, we as volunteer organisations should participate as much as possible. At the beginning, publicity was carried out on the first and second day of the (Lunar) New Year to make more people realise the severity of the epidemic and call for people to participate. [Int 6]
	As soon as the outbreak in January started, we considered that the outbreak was definitely different from the ordinary snowstorm and earthquake … [Int 10]
Volunteer Experience and Knowledge	Most members of our team are long-term volunteers. [Int 6]
	Many of us have experienced the Wenchuan earthquake in 2008. We all have experience. [Int 9]
	Many of them [volunteers] came out with me in 2005. At that time, everyone was in their 20s. By 2020 … our average age is around 35 or 40 years old. These people are relatively experienced. [Int 10]
	We have experienced a lot, including some events in China. I was in contact with these emergency-related things before, so I am relatively familiar with them … Many of our volunteers came from the Wenchuan earthquake in 2008. Some were medical staff, the disaster relief troops and township workers who had experienced SARS. [Int 10]
Volunteer Motivation	Since I'm a volunteer, I don't want anything in return, just everyone's safety. There is no subsidy from the government. [Int 2]
	The services from volunteers during the epidemic are selfless. People think it is worthwhile to make a contribution to their community or village as a volunteer. Our motives are unpaid and selfless. Everyone was very enthusiastic. [Int 3]
	We always wanted to contribute to the fight against the epidemic in our own way. When we learned about recruiting volunteers, we signed up without any hesitation. [Int 4]
	In the current epidemic, medical personnel are fighting on the front line, and many ordinary people in the rear are silently devoting their strength. We are happy and proud to be able to participate in such voluntary work, and hope that the epidemic will disappear as soon as possible. [Int 4]
	Everyone is selflessly devoted and asks nothing in return. [Int 8]
	We are also recruiting volunteers from our own group of friends. [Int 8]
	As ordinary people, they are willing to make a personal contribution to the society and the country. [Int 9]

While not all veteran volunteers had worked together before, many had done so locally or in previous emergencies. Several NPO leaders mentioned the experience of the Wenchuan earthquake and the SARS epidemic. This reflects findings from emergency management research that shared experience and previous interactions among crisis respondents can help build capacity to respond in an adaptive, coordinated manner (Comfort et al., 2001). One Zhejiang leader summarised this effectively, noting, "We worked with one heart" (Interview 13). Table 4.3 includes other quotes from the NPO leaders about the volunteers' motivations and efficacy.

Conclusion

This study shared insights from the first wave of the Covid-19 pandemic in China and offered lessons for future pandemics and other crises. Our research demonstrates how volunteers working in NPOs and state agencies can help communities meet urgent service demands during a crisis.

NPOs can mobilise and motivate volunteers by emphasising intangible incentives such as the ability to make a difference or have an impact by leveraging their professional skills to benefit their community. Our findings among early Covid-19 volunteers extend previous research regarding volunteer motivation to a new context of China's rapid response during an unprecedented pandemic. Our study found individuals were motivated to undertake community service through proximity and relevance of the crisis (Beyerlein & Sikkink, 2008; Gazley & Brudney, 2005) and social connections, especially bonding (versus bridging) ties (Rotolo & Berg, 2011). Community solidarity and duty played key roles in attracting volunteers (Finkelstein, 2010, Wilhelm & Bekkers, 2010), together with a belief in the ability to make an impact (Finolf, 2008; Wu et al., 2018). Prior experience and knowledge resources served as drivers and important success factors (Sundeen et al., 2007).

Our observations about volunteer motivation and experience align with the literature. The profile of the Zhejiang volunteers reflects the typology described by Van Eijk and Steen (2014), especially "semi-professional" and "network professional" volunteers. These volunteers enlist with the motivation to make a difference and achieve impact (rather than for social interaction, personal expression, or activism). As seen in Zhejiang, "semi-professional" volunteers can bring significant knowledge and experience to the task, especially coordinating efforts with public agencies. "Network professional" volunteers can bring service motivation, active experience, and empathy for client needs. Understanding these types of volunteers, their motivations, and their roles in delivering services is useful for continued efforts for recruitment and deployment to produce effective, professionalised services in a crisis.

Our study also demonstrated the value of technology. While recent studies highlight the role of digital technology in tracking and containment during global pandemics (Whitelaw et al., 2020), the rise of mobile technology also offers a promising and innovative approach to engaging volunteers in effective relief efforts. Mobile apps can overcome communication barriers (Weng et al., 2021), for instance, for volunteers who engage in emergency responses (McLennan et al., 2016) while broadcasting the volunteering experience via social media among family, friends, and peers.

As with all research, our study had limitations. The focus on a single country during a specific period of time limits our ability to make generalisations from the results. Going forward, future research should compare scenarios from several countries, ideally collecting data over multiple periods. In addition, longitudinal or multi-wave studies would help to unpack characteristics of the volunteer experience and factors influencing longer term motivation, engagement, involvement, and organisational commitment (Lapointe et al., 2019), especially as crises extend for months or years. Our findings offer a starting point from which to consider the potential of integrating volunteers into community responses in crisis situations, leveraging human capital and technology more systematically to meet societal needs.

References

Beyerlein, K., & Sikkink, D. (2008). Sorrow and solidarity: Why Americans volunteered for 9/11 relief efforts. *Social Problems, 55*(2), 190–215. 10.1525/sp.2008.55.2.190

Comfort, L.K., Sungy, Y., Johnson, D., & Dunn, M. (2001). Complex systems in crisis: Anticipation and resilience in dynamic environments. *Journal of Contingencies and Crisis Management, 9*(3), 144–158. 10.1111/1468-5973.00164

Einolf, C. (2008). Empathic concern and prosocial behaviors: A test of experimental results using survey data. *Social Science Research, 37*(4), 1267–1279. 10.1016/j.ssresearch.2007.06.003

Feduzi, A., Runde, J., & Schwarz, G. (2022). Unknowns, Black Swans, and bounded rationality in public organizations. *Public Administration Review, 82*(5), 958–963. 10.1111/puar.13522

Finkelstein, M. (2010). Individualism/collectivism: Implications for the volunteer process. *Social Behavior and Personality, 38*(4), 445–452. 10.2224/sbp.2010.38.4.445

Gazley, B., & Brudney, J.L. (2005). Volunteer involvement in local government after September 11: The continuing question of capacity. *Public Administration Review, 65*(2), 131–142. 10.1111/j.1540-6210.2005.00439.x

Harrison, D.A. (1995). Volunteer motivation and attendance decisions: Competitive theory testing in multiple samples from a homeless shelter. *Journal of Applied Psychology, 80*(3), 371–385. 10.1037/0021-9010.80.3.371

Hu, M. (2021). Making the state's volunteers in contemporary China. *Voluntas: International Journal of Voluntary and Nonprofit Organizations, 32*(6), 1375–1388. 10.1007/s11266-019-00190-9

Hu, M., Guo, C., & Bies, A. (2016). Termination of nonprofit alliances: Evidence from China. *Voluntas: International Journal of Voluntary and Nonprofit Organizations, 27*(5), 2490–2513. 10.1007/s11266-016-9698-z

Hustinx, L., Handy, F., & Cnaan, R. (2012). Student volunteering in China and Canada: Comparative perspectives. *Canadian Journal of Sociology, 37*(1), 55–83. 10.29173/cjs10363

Lapointe, É., Vandenberghe, C., Mignonac, K., Panaccio, A., Schwarz, G., Richebé, N., & Roussel, P. (2019). Development and validation of a commitment to organizational career scale: At the crossroads of organizational needs and individuals' career aspirations. *Journal of Occupational and Organizational Psychology, 92*(4), 897–930. 10.1111/joop.12273

Maher, C.S., Huong, T., & Hindery, A. (2020). Fiscal responses to COVID-19: Evidence from local governments and nonprofits. *Public Administration Review, 80*(4), 644–650. 10.1111/puar.13238

McDonald, S. (2009). Changing climate, changing minds: Applying the literature on media effects, public opinion, and the issue-attention cycle to increase public understanding of climate change. *International Journal of Sustainability Communication, 4*, 45–63.

McLennan, B., Whittaker, J., & Handmer, J. (2016). The changing landscape of disaster volunteering: Opportunities, responses and gaps in Australia. *Natural Hazards, 84*(3), 2031–2048. 10.1007/s11069-016-2532-5

Nesbit, R., Christensen, R.K., & Brudney, J.L. (2018). The limits and possibilities of volunteering: A framework for explaining the scope of volunteer involvement in public and nonprofit organizations. *Public Administration Review, 78*(4), 502–513. 10.1111/puar.12894

Rotolo, T., & Berg, (2011). In times of need: An examination of emergency preparedness and disaster relief service volunteers. *Nonprofit and Voluntary Sector Quarterly, 40*(4), 740–750. 10.1177/0899764010369179

Schwarz, G., Newman, A., Yu, J., & Michaels, V. (2021). Psychological entitlement and organizational citizenship behaviors: The roles of employee involvement climate and affective organizational commitment. *The International Journal of Human Resource Management*, 10.1080/09585192.2021.1962388

Stukas, A.A., Hoye, R., Nicholson, M., Brown, K.M., & Aisbett, L. (2016). Motivations to volunteer and their associations with volunteers' well-being. *Nonprofit and Voluntary Sector Quarterly, 45*(1), 112–132. 10.1177/0899764014561122

Sundeen, R., Raskoff, S., & Garcia, C. (2007). Differences in perceived barriers to volunteering to formal organizations: Lack of time versus lack of interest. *Nonprofit Management and Leadership, 17*(3), 279–300. 10.1002/nml.150

van Eijk, C.J.A., & Steen, T.P.S. (2014). Why people co-produce: Analysing citizens' perceptions on co-planning engagement in health care services. *Public Management Review, 16*(3), 358–382. 10.1080/14719037.2013.841458

Wang, C., & Wu, X. (2014). Volunteers' motivation, satisfaction, and management in large-scale events: An empirical test from the 2010 Shanghai World Expo. *Voluntas: International Journal of Voluntary and Nonprofit Organizations, 25*(3), 754–771. 10.1007/s11266-013-9350-0

Weng, S., Schwarz, G., Schwarz, S., & Hardy, B. (2021). A framework for government response to social media participation in public policy making: Evidence from China. *International Journal of Public Administration, 44*(16), 1424–1434. 10.1080/01900692.2020.1852569

Whitelaw, S., Mamas, M.A., Topol, E., & Van Spall, G.C. (2020). Applications of digital technology in COVID-19 pandemic planning and response. *The Lancet, 2*(8), E435–E440. 10.1016/S2589-7500(20)30142-4

Wilhelm, M., & Bekkers, R. (2010). Helping behavior, dispositional empathic concern and the principle of care. *Social Psychology Quarterly, 73*(1), 11–32. 10.1177/0190272510361435

Wilson, J. (2012). Volunteerism research: A review essay. *Nonprofit and Voluntary Sector Quarterly, 41*(2), 176–212. 10.1177/0899764011434558

Wu, Y.L., Shao, B., Newman, A., & Schwarz, G. (2021). Crisis leadership: A review and future research agenda. *The Leadership Quarterly, 32*(6), 101518. 10.1016/j.leaqua.2021.101518

Wu, Z., Zhao, R., Zhang, X., & Liu, F. (2018). The impact of social capital on volunteering and giving: Evidence from urban China. *Nonprofit and Voluntary Sector Quarterly, 47*(6), 1201–1222. 10.1177/0899764018784761

Zhang, S. et al. (2020). COVID-19 containment: China provides important lessons for global response. *Frontiers of Medicine, 14*(2), 215–219. 10.1007/s11684-020-0766-9

5 Grassroots Movements and Covid-19 in Buenos Aires. Vital Networking and Social Media in Times of Crisis

Victoria D'hers

Introduction

After two years marked by dystopia made true, how do social changes and new forms of representation originate, in the context of a pandemic and the so-called public policy of ASPO Aislamiento Social Preventivo y Obligatorio (*Preventive and Mandatory Social Confinement*), the main public policy in Argentina during Covid-19? The diagnoses of the crisis will determine the "exits" and solutions: what policies will be adopted to revive devastated economies? In the Global South, it is likely that these policies will be linked to multiple forms of extractivist practices. In 2022, the "new normal" seems to be a bad copy of the old one, even though, as many social movements state, normality was the problem. The world system has strengthened its mechanisms of intercontinental exploitation, both of bodies and the earth, and inequalities are being reflected even more clearly.

On the one hand, at the environmental level, there was no cessation or decrease in pollution and environmental suffering, as predicted in March 2020, but an increase. Regarding social relations, global solidarity did not take the place of competition at the level that was expected at the beginning of 2020. The excessive enrichment of certain corporations and the extreme impoverishment of a large number of people throughout the planet were remarkable. The numbers of people experiencing poverty continue to increase as a global phenomenon (Oxfam, 2020). By the end of 2021, the richest 10% of the population (further enriched during the periods of lockdown) concentrated 56% of the wealth and the poorest 50% had 8% of the income (Pellecier & Grasso, 2021). This is recognisably a problem for sustainable development (United Nations, 2021). In the case of Argentina, 37.3% of the population was poor, according to data from the INDEC (National Institute of Statistics and Census) corresponding to the second half of 2021. Even though public policies were generated (like the IFE, *Ingreso Federal de Emergencia,* Federal Emergency Income), the basic everyday life needs were not fulfilled by the local state.

On the other hand, in addition to reviewing the structural level of this new (old) normality, it is important to analyse the *interstitial* level (Scribano, 2014, 2020; D'hers, 2022a); the spaces through which indifference opens cracks and

DOI: 10.4324/9781003301905-6

the networks, which guarantee daily survival, are strengthened. In short, interstitial practices imply love, happiness, and reciprocity. This reciprocity reassures the potency of the collective, being and reaffirming "us" as a group, rather than acting as individuals. As it has been observed in the field of grassroots movements, the social bonds that arise and are strengthened in the form of a vital and vitalising network appear as a central part of the *social sensibilities*, which pulsate daily to resist the iteration of suffering.

From here arises the question about the social sensitivities of popular neighbourhood movements with a strong influence in social networks in times of lockdown. In the midst of the coronavirus crisis, the main ways of prevention were hygiene and social distancing measures. However, since the beginning of the pandemic, structural problems – which were pre-existing – became evident, such as the lack of drinking water or overcrowded houses. Basic care was impossible. Hence, the question that emerges refers to the ways in which this reality was made visible and interpreted by people living in these conditions, particularly from an intersectional perspective.

This chapter analyses the role of social grassroots organisations, drawing upon the sociology of bodies, emotions, and social sensibilities. Specifically, observing La Garganta Poderosa[1] – the social media network of La Poderosa movement – and how it was efficient in both communicating this crisis to a broader public, even drawing attention from the local and national state, and generating a common feeling of the power of grassroots movements. Specifically, how did more people realise that their suffering was not individual, but caused by social structures? And further, what was the role of social media in this context? In this chapter, I present some preliminary reflections based on qualitative methodology, particularly digital ethnography of the movement's social media, and participant observation in assemblies and women's meetings during 2021 in a neighbourhood in the south of Buenos Aires. The order is as follows: first, I discuss the methodology applied here; then, a conceptual synthesis of the sociology of bodies and emotions as tools to understand the contemporary social structuring of social sensibilities. Finally, I propose a preliminary analysis of what was published by La Garganta Poderosa – a social collective organisation pre-existing the pandemic – in its social networks related to the pandemic, to visualise its role during this time of exception. This study seeks to understand in what ways these spaces gained importance (even more than they previously had) in times of global crisis.

Methodological Approach

The present study is based on an approach to the online activity of a social organisation. It is based on a qualitative approach, which seeks to reconstruct social sensibilities; specifically, a digital ethnography (Ardevol & Gómez-Cruz, 2014).

The data corpus comprises the public social media posts made by La Garganta Poderosa, related to the Covid-19 pandemic and its effects in slums.

An investigation of the central subjects was carried out, identifying key points in relation to social sensibilities and the pandemic. The study also included references to participant observation in weekly cultural meetings organised by the movement, with women from a neighbourhood in the south of Buenos Aires, since May 2021. The objective of the chapter is to critically analyse the online data of a social movement, which reveals how social sensibilities were referred to during Covid-19, and the social suffering in this reality.

Social Sensibilities as a Lens in the Pandemic

Beyond the fact that social sciences are defined as going through a *sensory turn* (Howes, 2014) and *bodily/corporeal turn* (Scribano, 2012), the need to understand sensibilities and to reflect upon its social configuration is indisputable. Emotions, bodies, and social structuring are knotted and co-constitute each other. Moreover, in this context of *new normality*, the multiple normalisations that sustain the social as the "only possible way of life" became palpable as never before.

The politics of sensibilities are understood as "the set of cognitive-affective social practices tending to the production, management and reproduction of horizons of action, disposition and cognition" (Scribano, 2017b, p. 244). More specifically, within a sociology of bodies/emotions it is understood that:

> the image body is an indicator of the process of how 'I see that I am seen'. From its side, the body skin indicates the process of how I 'naturally sense' the world, and the body movement is the bodily inscription of the possibilities of action. The interactions among body image, body skin and body movement are taken as signallers (indicators) of social domination and as locators of class situation.
>
> (Scribano, 2012, p. 101)

Thus, the analysis of "social pain" and its multiple manifestations has been proposed (D'hers, 2013; D'hers & Cervio, 2019; Cervio, Lisdero & D'hers, 2020). As a part of such a phenomenon, the feminisation of poverty is undisputed and must be considered (D'hers, 2022a, 2022b).

How, then does intersectionality reveal and contribute to the explanation of social pain? The African-American theorist Kimberlé Crenshaw developed the concept of intersectionality in 1989, within a critical dialogue in the feminist movement[2]. In the context of law studies, she challenged the legal landscape, from feminist and racial perspectives, observing how judicial measures in the labour context aggravated discrimination. Then, in 2002, the UN recognised the "intersectional nature" of discrimination. The intersectional perspective allows us then to sharpen our understanding of discrimination, as we discern how these women *embody* the different levels of violence, and how these levels are raised. Far from the idea of a simple "addition", ethnicity, class, nationality, and the associated violence intersect and enhance their effects.

Now, in relation to care and caring practices, women are usually the ones who undertake them. This was accentuated during the pandemic, exacerbating the social suffering and pain involved. In fact, Latin America is the most unsafe region for women, who are the victims of gender violence and feminicide (Svampa, 2020). As mentioned, the pandemic operated as a magnifying glass (D'hers, 2022a) displaying more clearly than usual certain "mechanisms of social bearability" (Scribano, 2012, p. 100) in operation and reproduction. At the same time, it is also a magnifying glass for these interstitial practices that make *networks* and social *bonds*; instances where feminist collectives have radical importance. Understanding the configuration of social sensibilities is the key to breaking apart the multiple facets of social domination. This domination operates in daily life, becomes flesh, is embodied, then being produced and reproduced. Being part of social configuration, it is lived as intimate and personal. So this involves evidencing and problematising how sensitivity is embodied and "created", making visible how an individual's *perceptual frame* becomes a node of daily systemic violence (Bourdieu, 2010).

Finally, it is also possible to observe the emergence of other sensibilities, amid a renewed capitalism defined by its permanent ongoing metamorphosis. Whether linked to housing (D'hers, 2022a), to other modes of agricultural production (Veiguela & D'hers, 2021), or the present writing that seeks to make visible daily violence but also interstitial practices. In this framework, I raise the possibility of filial love as a way out, linked to practices of happiness, hope and reciprocity (Scribano, 2017b, 2020), understanding that #*lasalidaescolectiva* (#thewayoutiscollective), as will be discussed next.

Communication Networks: Safety and Power Networks

Since 2020, poverty and inequality have worsened worldwide. There are several works related to the problem of Covid-19 in underserved neighbourhoods and precarious settlements in Latin America. For example, there is information regarding actions of "solidarity and empathy" on the website Synergies for Solidarity (www.synergiesforsolidarity.org). Also in this vein, Ortiz and Di Virgilio (2020), writing about Argentina, state that "the slogan 'stay at home' is difficult to follow in conditions in which the access to decent housing is not guaranteed"[3].

In the same way, the centrality of territorial actions and the importance of local practices from pre-existing collectives that guaranteed the possibility of feeding large numbers of people in marginalised neighbourhoods became clear to society. In the case of La Garganta Poderosa, its importance has been observed in the distribution of donations received during the pandemic (food, cleaning products, and alcohol gel). Also, it provided essential emotional support, offering a meeting place and carrying out weekly visits to neighbours to ensure their safety.

La Poderosa is a movement and an organisation, which is present in several countries in Latin America and the Caribbean. They have Assemblies in Argentina, Bolivia, Brazil, Chile, Colombia, Mexico, Paraguay, Peru, and Uruguay. Its logo and name are due to the nickname of the motorcycle on which Ernesto "Che" Guevara travelled the continent in the 1950s. The organisation was founded in 2004, a response to the social, economic, and political crises in Argentina of the years from 2001 (the famous political demand "*Que se vayan todos*" – "Make them all go!": a general public demand that all politicians quit their jobs, making the representational crisis evident. This is an historical moment, when the so-called cacerolazos emerged)[4].

Then, in 2011 La Garganta Poderosa (LGP), its magazine in print format emerged to counter the hegemonic discourse that circulates in the mass media and stigmatises those who live in slums:

> This publication was born as a product of the articulation of neighbourhood assemblies to build a way of organisation that had nothing to do either with welfare or with benefactor hands, but with our own logic, without commercial advertising, or official guidelines, as a way to face problems that traverse our neighbourhoods. One of these problems has to do with the stigmatisation of the neighbourhoods by the mainstream media.
>
> (Porritelli, 2013, p. 1)

Mazzini and Ficoseco (2020) show that social media reinforce circulating social images. Thus, the LGP social media seek to establish their own view, manifested from the marginalised neighbourhoods and making explicit the need to break the silence about their day-to-day life. This message is clear in the emblematic covers of the magazine on which celebrities (musicians, actors, sportsmen like Lionel Messi and Diego Maradona) appear in shouting gestures:

> La Garganta was born from the cry of the soul, from the bowels of popular power. Maybe it vomits, maybe it sings, maybe it laughs, maybe it spits. But it's going to scream, La Garganta is going to scream (…) These are times of new voices and we are going to fight on our own, as always, with photography bullets and cannon pens, now organised from our place in the world.
>
> (LGP First editorial, cited in González, 2013, p. 11)

The magazine is run by cooperatives of different neighbourhoods and cities, which belong to the LP movement. It relies on an "us" and is based on a necessary resistance to establish "a place in the world". This collective sense is reinforced and redefined in the heat of reality, as we will see in the next section. The magazine is a result of civil society organisation, promoting social change. These experiences are referred to as "social or civic journalism", which "transforms the citizen into an active agent of journalistic processes" (Pagani & Gómez, 2020, p. 63). Synthetically,

1) it focuses its theme on the problems of marginalised neighbourhoods, also called "villas" (slums), 2) is carried out entirely by residents of those neighbourhoods and 3) the way of approaching the subjects is made from the perspective and discursive style of its own protagonists, generating a break in the graphic and visual languages characteristic of traditional media.

(Pagani & Gómez, 2020, p. 63)

These media constitute claims against the gaze of the stigma of the "negro de mierda" ("black shit"). In a country where there is a lack of recognition of the importance of its indigenous past, and a whitening of its history, racist practices are a daily problem. In response to this, this magazine deals with the identity of the neighbourhood, makes the aforementioned "us" evident, drawing attention to the problems of the material conditions of existence; most of all, seeking to capture the achievements of the neighbourhoods. Both the print magazine and the social media posts try to show the problems, but they also show how collective organisation allows the people from the neighbourhood "to achieve great things and transform everything that an absent or exclusive State does not deal with" (LGP First Editorial, 2011). The feeling of "kinship" and community is present in the statements of the members of the magazine, who seek to build *from the collective*. This is key to counter social exclusion. Then, in dialogue with the previously referenced "filial love", we now observe certain practices linked to love as a mobilising energy and power.

Some Lines of Action in Social Media

As described on its Instagram profile, La Garganta Poderosa is a "Magazine of *Villera*[5] culture, the literary arm of the La Poderosa movement" (La Garganta Poderosa, n.d.). Its Instagram has, in April 2022, 519,000 followers, and its Facebook has 711,988. This section aims to examine how sensitivities were shaped during the pandemic, in this group and in relation to its followers. The problems of exclusion are the predominant subject in all the stories and interviews. Themes addressed include police repression, gender violence, sexual and gender diversity, precarious and unsanitary conditions in homes and neighbourhoods, immigration, the way in which the media show poverty or neighbourhoods, work, and rights in general (Pagani & Gómez, 2020). Considering these subjects from an intersectional perspective, we see once again the overlap of violence in the neighbourhoods, marked by poverty and violation. Within a social movement of this kind of neighbourhood, intersecting inequalities of class, gender, and ethnicity are evident.

In the analysis below, I highlight the conceptual points linked to the production of social sensitivities. I use italics for excerpts from publications.

In the first place, during the pandemic this communication space emerged as a platform to denounce the real impossibility of carrying out the basic practices of prevention of Covid-19. At the end of April 2020, several publications sounded the alarm on the arrival of the virus in different towns in the city of Buenos Aires, insisting on the impossibility of confinement:

> *"We have just confirmed two new cases of Covid-19 in another Buenos Aires popular neighbourhood, where the authorities have already recognised that many cannot comply with isolation at home, where the only provision of the City has been to promote community confinement, where the virus is already a reality inhabiting the same community and where the officials of the Ministry of Health of the City are assuming that they only have at their disposal the 300 beds of the Curas Villeros* [Neighbourhood Priests]*".*
>
> (La Poderosa, 2020a)

In times of the so-called new normal, the writers in these media defined the threshold of the bearable for the neighbourhoods, manifesting the evident and also invisible: the impossibility of sustaining basic hygiene and distancing measures recommended incessantly in all the media. In May 2020, cases were on the rise, and services were deficient:

> *We have been without water in the neighbourhood during the last four days, with 13 confirmed cases of coronavirus. How do you want us to comply with all the prevention and hygiene measures? In my family this impacts much harder because we are six people, and four are part of the at-risk population. We live in overcrowded conditions, which complicates the care we take with Guada, my daughter, who was diagnosed with West Syndrome and Aicardi Syndrome when she was 5 months old. She suffers refractory convulsions, and she has 34 points for a scoliosis surgery that worsens because of humidity. Guada cries, screams, is constantly sad, with dark circles under her eyes, and her convulsions are more frequent.*
>
> (La Garganta Poderosa, 2020a)

The daily suffering, accentuated by housing and health precarity was exacerbated in a context of permanent threat of contagion. Emotions of sadness were accentuated by the impossibility of sustaining care. The mentioned *body skin* suffers and is marked by each day of suffering. Ramona Medina became an emblem of both the struggle and resistance of the neighbourhood, as well as the neglect and abandonment by the state. Founder of the Woman's House[6] in 2018, she died in May 2020, at a time when she was highlighting the lack of drinking water during the pandemic (Cf. Post from May 22nd – #Ramonanosecalla – #RamonaDoesn'tStaySilent, La Garganta Poderosa, 2020b). She is referred to as the inspiration, a "semilla" (seed) for the generation of new spaces and social dining rooms in various neighbourhoods and settlements in the provinces (it is usual that the communal spaces have the name of their martyrs and victims).

Towards the middle of May 2020, the LGP publications on Instagram highlighted the increasing number of cases in the neighbourhoods. This fact was "silenced" by the official media and authorities in a post from May 11th, 2020: "Silence is never health". In the post, it reads:

> *"Senior citizens are an at-risk group, thanks to the decision of coronavirus. But poor people are an at-risk group through the decision of who 'urbanised', provided no basic urban services, or water: 373 cases in Villa 31 [a name of a neighbourhood]; 120 in 1-11-14 [a name of a neighbourhood]; 519 in popular neighbourhoods of CABA, Buenos Aires City. More than 500 cases of coronavirus in Buenos Aires' slums. Silence is never health. Now Rodriguez Larreta [Governor of Buenos Aires] mumbles in front of Tenenbaum [a journalist], to yield our legal demands arguing that he does not do 'cheap politics', as if it was not cheap politics to pay in order to make poor people invisible, silence pacts on entire districts and talk about 'one city'".*
>
> (La Garganta Poderosa, 2020c)

Besides, within the centrality of the collective, during this time, bonds with other organisations solidified. For example, donations of vegetables and fruits were received from the UTT collective (Union of Workers of the Earth) (La Poderosa, 2020b). People talk about a "chain of humanity": *In Villa Azul, in Zavaleta, or anywhere on the planet, the community at the service of the community. #ContagiáSolidaridad* (La Garganta Poderosa, 2020d).

Another main point to observe is how the environmental question and the impact of pollution on bodies is treated, always through the class perspective:

> *In one of the provinces with the highest soybean production in the country, where thousands of hectares are used ceaselessly for planting, we continue to suffer the reality that poisons us: fumigation with pesticides. Yes, although 107 of these toxic chemicals used to kill insects, weeds, and all kinds of fungi are forbidden in the world according to the World Health Organisation and the Food and Agriculture Organisation of the United Nations, since their consequences are harmful to the environment and people's health. In Entre Ríos, we have suffered for a long time: "I am 50 years old and I live with my 91 years old mother, my 70 years old partner, and my son, who is 24; our house has been sprayed repeatedly since 2017 and, although it seems incredible, in the middle of quarantine they sprayed us again!", says Lidia Moreira, a resident of the sixth district of Gualeguay.*
>
> (La Garganta Poderosa, 2020e)

In April 2020, in the middle of a lockdown requiring full isolation and restriction of all activity, the state established certain "productive activities" such as agriculture as essential activities. With the expression "to spray", besides the literality of the term ("pulverizar" means "to spray" in Spanish), Lidia seemed to also refer to the feeling of "being made dust", destroyed by that system of exploitation that will not stop in the middle of a worldwide pause. Thus, these examples establish the certainty of the solidarity networks as "safety nets" (*redes de contención* in Spanish):

Weaving the nets that sustain us every day, walking these steps with dignity as a guide, fighting against the isolation of the lack of communication, guaranteeing education in our neighbourhoods, being realistic when we are dreaming of the impossible, shouting loudly against the inadmissible, making our voices multiply, knowing that we have you, we stand on our hands to uproot so much inequality.

(La Garganta Poderosa, 2020f)

Another central objective of social media is the role of the *Villero* Observatory, where they collect their own data, in contrast to what is reported by the official statistics – not only about the pandemic but statistics in general. This shows the central role they have as spokespersons and representatives of what happens in the neighbourhoods, in the words of those who live there. For example, in another publication, official statistics from the INDEC (the National Institute of Statistics and Census) on poverty, are discussed:

Clear estimates: inequality is maintained: According to the INDEC, a family of 5 people needs $71,899 [Argentinian pesos] not to be poor and $30,726 not to be indigent. In our neighbourhoods, that limit is a bit far away: according to our Villero Observatory, any of our families has an average income of $23, 750, equivalent to a third of the Basic Products Parcel, which puts us $6,976 below the indigence line and $48,149 below the poverty line. How do we survive day by day? Fathers and mothers in different neighbourhoods of the country usually have only a cup of mate cocido [a typical tea made with a herb called yerbamate] to give as a plate of food to their children. This is the daily struggle that we live in poor neighbourhoods, condemned to neglect and abandonment, without even being able to appeal the sentence: this is how we survive, under the line of indigence.

(La Garganta Poderosa, 2020g)

Here is a clear and crude exposition of the problem of hunger, once again. The urgency is indisputable, and it is clear that the non-resolution of this issue does not impact only on the present, but above all on future possibilities. Hunger functions as the ultimate restriction on the possibilities of thought and autonomy, both regarding the possibility to move and to think (Scribano, 2012). During the pandemic, there was a general recognition of those who supported the popular kitchens. As I stated elsewhere (D'hers, 2022a), this was not limited to the times of confinement, but that time of exception put a magnifying glass on what was already happening. One year after the beginning of the Covid-19 pandemic and already with an advanced vaccination campaign in the country, this issue became clear. It turned into a claim for vaccines for community cooks, demanding that they be considered as *essential workers*, as doctors and nurses were. Here, at the level of communication and impact, the magazine relies on art, entertainment, and cultural figures, as it is seen in an image which it circulated which depicted the Mexican singer Julieta Venegas (La Garganta Poderosa, 2020h)[7].

One year into the pandemic, the issue was already clear, and the experiences were overwhelming: the need of solidarity networks was evident, and the work of the residents of the *villas* was key for the daily functioning of community spaces. The weekly meetings guaranteed care, and the work of the women who supported the kitchens was and is of great importance. A radical transformation occurred: the fear of contagion of the virus turned into #transmitsolidarity (*#contagiasolidaridad*).

In addition, the hashtag #transmitconnectivity (*#contagiaconectividad*) referred to campaigns for internet access, another scarce resource that became vital. Thanks to these "safety nets", daily survival[8], as it is called, is possible: *"Safety nets. Hey, Zuckerberg, here are the networks that work"* (La Garganta Poderosa, 2021b).

It should be noted that the Poderosa collective is present all over the country, strengthening its voice and demands. In a post from Tucumán province, known as The Republic Garden, the name was changed to The Hunger of the Republic. This "garden" is ironically one of the provinces with the highest poverty rates:

> *The hunger of the republic. There is hunger, and at this point we don't know what else to do. That's why, with an empty belly and anguish pierced in our throats, we shout. At every corner of our country, the food demand does not stop increasing and, in the province of Tucumán, we are in a dire situation: we currently put our soul in seven popular kitchens and seven 'merenderos' (places where children may eat some snacks in the afternoon) to guarantee more than 7,000 daily food dishes without State contribution. Every day, more families are coming, arriving up to four hours earlier so as not to miss out on the food distribution, and we still have no solutions from the provincial government.*
>
> (La Garganta Poderosa, 2021c)

Finally, regarding feminism and feminist networks (which would take a whole chapter), the care provided by the residents is not only related to food, but also to the daily monitoring of people and their domestic situation. This care which caught public media during the pandemic, is transversal and transcends the situation of 2020 (D'hers, 2022a).

Final Thoughts

It is 2022. The conversations no longer refer only to the numbers of deceased or hospitalised but are about vaccines and what number of doses each one has. We cannot yet account for the deep levels at which Covid-19 affected us both personally and socially, but we are moving forward. After the worst, apparently, the effects remain. The visible ones, and above all, those that will go on across generations. No one yet knows the full impact of this global pandemic, prolonged in time, unprecedented, and as variable and uncertain as it is threatening.

At a juncture of post-pandemic crisis, seemingly the heyday of the control society, how do changes emerge at the societal and microsocial levels? What practices do we observe? The social sciences have an important role to play in this dispute over the meanings of the crisis. The significance and sensations that become embodied and make calluses.

Considering the context of the pandemic, and strict confinement in the first months, especially in Buenos Aires, this visibility of the role of social groups and organisations proves to be of interest: La Garganta Poderosa's social networks functioned to monitor cases and the progress of the virus. In the absence of records and tests in the underserved neighbourhoods, they reported on the numbers of Covid-19 patients in their publications. In addition, they accentuated and made visible *#lasalidaescolectiva* (#theexitiscollective), insisting that *#nadiesesalvasolo* (nobody is saved on their own).

This social pain is not new (D'hers, 2022a). Before Covid-19, there was a clear conviction:

> *La Garganta Poderosa is born as a result of the conviction of the people about the 'power to change the world, to make us happy, transform tears into smiles, generate a new reality within this reality'.*
>
> ("Words that break stigmas", published in the magazine, extracted from Gonzalez, 2013, p. 8)

How was happiness defined before, how it is redefined in this new normal? What role does reciprocity play? Just as we revised the notion of essentiality, and the delimitation of "essential activities", what parameters will we build to build this culture of care and this new reality? What place do women have, when they meet and make explicit that violence is not due to individual circumstances? And what role do social networks play in this context: in what ways do they collectively deconstruct and reconstruct subjectivity?

Finally, we consider it relevant to remember that these pages are part of an elaboration which is always situated; the creation of theory is always an experience, and above all an experience of listening rather than speaking in the name of other people.

Notes

1 Literally translated from Spanish, this means *The Powerful Throat*, indicating also a powerful and loud voice.
2 In this line, authors like Sumi Cho, Kimberlé Crenshaw and Leslie McCall (2013) defend that intersectionality is an analytical sensitivity, a way of thinking and analysing. Based on this premise, the authors state that "'an intersectional analysis is not settled by the fact of using the word *intersectionality* into a text, but it is a way of thinking of sameness, difference and their relationship with power'" (Rodó Zárate, 2021, p. 32). Patricia Hill Collins (2019) and Clorinda Matto de Turner, among others, also understand that intersectional oppression is a 'matrix of oppression', and that this analytical sensitivity was

already present before the explanation of the term. NOTE: The author of this chapter translated into English all the passages extracted from references in other languages.

3 For a view of the pandemic and the health system in Argentina, see Testa (2020).

4 After years of an unreal convertibility of the national peso to US dollar (1 dollar = 1 peso), and the impoverishment of large numbers of working- and middle-class people due to the closure of enterprises and factories, the economic crisis erupted at the end of 2001. The banks closed, and the President Fernando De La Rua had to flee the government, as an example of the general lack of political trust. Then the *cacerolazo* emerged: a way of social protest which gathered mainly urban middle-class people onto the streets making noise with their kitchen pans (*cacerolas*), reclaiming their right to withdraw their money from banks and in US currency. This translated into political crisis, with a succession of several presidents in only one month.

5 *Villera* relates to slums, as stated before. We choose to use the Spanish word since the aim of this media is to give value to this specific reality and culture.

6 A social space created by the residents, for women to refer to in case of need, or if exposed to violent situations.

7 As I indicated at the beginning of the section, this 'us' is reclaimed, and defined as that 'us' of perseverance, embodied suffering, and it also relates to celebrities and icons. Another example is the relevance given to Diego A. Maradona: *"You made the whole word know all the pains we suffer. You are the 'villa' in your own flesh"* (La Garganta Poderosa, 2021a).

8 Eventhough there is no sufficient space to analyse such big issue, the role of LGP to seek, mourn and remember numerous disappeared or killed girls is worthy of mention. The collective embodies the absence of women and girls who are still waiting to find those who perpetrated brutal rapes, most of the time within their own families, and which are normalised.

References

Ardévol, E. & Gómez-Cruz, E. (2014). Digital ethnography and media practices. In Valdivia, A.N. (Ed.), *The international encyclopedia of media studies* (1st. Ed., Vol. VII). John Wiley & Sons.

Bourdieu, P. (2010 [1980]). *El Sentido Práctico.* Siglo Veintiuno Editores.

Cervio, A.L., Lisdero, P. & D'hers, V. (2020). "Cuerpos precarios": Habitar, respirar y trabajar en el Sur Global. Una mirada desde la sociología de los cuerpos/emociones. *Empiria. Revista de Metodología de Ciencias Sociales, 47,* 43–63. URL: http://revistas.uned. es/index.php/empiria/article/view/27424; DOI: 10.5944/empiria.47.2020.27424

D'hers, V. (2022a). Cuando la pandemia es un peligro más. El rol vital de colectivos feministas en barrios marginados. In Gravante, T. & Regalado (Eds.), *Alternativas, resistencias y auto-cuidado colectivo frente al COVID-19 y a la crisis socioambiental.* (pp. 209–228). UNAM. ISBN 978-607-30-5910-7. URL: https://www.ceiich.unam.mx/0/50NovLib.php?id=750

D'hers, V. (2022b). "Yo no salgo, estoy encerrada en mi casa." Espacio urbano y encierro desde narrativas sensibles pre pandemia. In De Sena, A. (Ed.), *Sensibilidades, Subjetividades y Pobreza.* GT CLACSO. In print.

D'hers, V. (2013). Encarnando la necesidad: Cuerpos, espacios y habitus en dos barrios del conurbano, Provincia de Buenos Aires, Argentina. *Revista INTERSTICIOS, 7*(1), 115–130. ISSN 1887-3898. URL: http://www.intersticios.es/article/view/11256

D'hers, V. & Cervio, A.L. (2019). Dolor social, conflictividad y pobreza: Un abordaje desde las experiencias de inmigrantes limítrofes en la Ciudad de Buenos Aires. *Digithum, 23,* 1–13. Universitat Oberta de Catalunya and Universidad de Antioquia. DOI: 10.7238/d.v0i23.3142

González, V. (2013). *Palabras que abren puertas: Una lectura sobre la experiencia cooperativa de la revista barrial "La Garganta Poderosa", desde la perspectiva de la Comunicación Popular de Paulo Freire*. Córdoba, Argentina: [Conference Presentation] IV Encuentro Panamericano de Comunicación. URL: https://www.publicacioncompanam2013.eci.unc.edu.ar/files/companam/ponencias/Producci%C3%B3n%20en%20medios%20alternativos/-Unlicensed-PMA-y-PS.Gonz%C3%A1lez-Ver%C3%B3nica-Andrea.pdf

Hill Collins, P. & Blige (2019). *Interseccionalidad*. Ediciones Morata.

Howes, D. (2014). El creciente campo de los Estudios Sensoriales. *Revista Latinoamericana de Estudios sobre Cuerpos, Emociones y Sociedad - RELACES*, *15*, 10–26. URL: http://www.relaces.com.ar/index.php/relaces/article/view/319/314

La Garganta Poderosa [@lagargantapoderosa]. (n.d.). Posts [Instagram profile]. Retrieved from https://www.instagram.com/lagargantapoderosa/

La Garganta Poderosa [@lagargantapoderosa]. (2021a, June 22). Todos los dolores que sufrimos, hiciste que los conociera el mundo entero. Sos la villa en carne viva, #GraciasDiego [Instagram photo]. Retrieved from https://www.instagram.com/p/CQbwRqxg2rU/

La Garganta Poderosa [@lagargantapoderosa]. (2021b, October 5). Redes de contención. Che, Zuckerberg, acá están las redes que funcionan. [Instagram video]. Retrieved from https://www.instagram.com/p/CQbwRqxg2rU/

La Garganta Poderosa [@lagargantapoderosa]. (2021c, October 22). "El hambre de la república". Hay hambre, y a esta altura del partido no sabemos qué más hacer. Por eso, con la panza vacía y la angustia atravesada en la garganta, gritamos igual. En cada rincón de nuestro país, la demanda …" [Instagram video]. Retrieved from https://www.instagram.com/p/CVWHHsHBMjy/

La Garganta Poderosa [@lagargantapoderosa]. (2020a, April 29). Así no se puede vivir. Por Ramona Medina, vecina del sector Bajo autopista, Villa 31. Hace 4 días estamos sin agua en el barrio, aún con 13 casos confirmados de coronavirus. ¿Cómo pretenden que cumplamos todas las medidas de prevención … [Instagram photo]. Retrieved from https://www.instagram.com/p/B_lMBONgGMb/

La Garganta Poderosa [@lagargantapoderosa]. (2020b, May 22). Cuando la injusticia nos duele, cuando el cinismo nos daña, cuando la pauta nos censura, cuando la bronca nos atraganta, cuando la realidad nos desmorona … Seguimos en pie, gritando, gracias a la garganta de Ramona [Instagram photo]. Retrieved from https://www.instagram.com/p/CAf1AdMgiym/

La Garganta Poderosa [@lagargantapoderosa]. (2020c, May 11). El silencio nunca es salud. Ahora, Rodríguez Larreta balbucea frente a Tenembaum, para poder esquivar nuestras denuncias aludiendo que no hace "politiquería", como si no fuera politiquería pagar para invisibilizar a los pobres, tender pactos de silencio sobre barrios enteros … [Instagram photo]. Retrieved from https://www.instagram.com/p/CADx1MhA35o/

La Garganta Poderosa [@lagargantapoderosa]. (2020d, June 1). Cadena de humanidad. En Villa Azul, en Zavaleta, o en cualquier parte del planeta, la comunidad al servicio de la comunidad. #ContagiáSolidaridad [Instagram video]. Retrieved from https://www.instagram.com/p/CA3shTSA7wd/

La Garganta Poderosa [@lagargantapoderosa]. (2020e, June 13). Aislamiento Tóxico. En una de las provincias con mayor producción sojera del país, donde miles de hectáreas son utilizadas sin descanso para la siembra, seguimos sufriendo la realidad que nos envenena: Las fumigaciones con agrotóxicos. Sí, aunque 107 de estas … [Instagram photo]. Retrieved from https://www.instagram.com/p/CBY7zDXAxFM/

La Garganta Poderosa [@lagargantapoderosa]. (2020f, August 12). Redes de contención. Tejiendo las redes que nos sostienen cada día, caminando estos pasos con la dignidad como guía, combatiendo el aislamiento de la incomunicación, garantizando en nuestras barriadas la educación, siendo realistas al soñar lo imposible, gritando bien fuerte … [Instagram photo]. Retrieved from https://www.instagram.com/p/CDyrxPsjM8w/

La Garganta Poderosa [@lagargantapoderosa]. (2020g, September 29). Cuentas claras: Conservan la desigualdad. Según el INDEC, una familia de 5 integrantes necesita $71.899 para no ser pobre y $30.726 para no ser indigente. En nuestros barrios, ese límite nos queda un poco lejos: según nuestro Observatorio … [Instagram photo]. Retrieved from https://www.instagram.com/p/CUaR7iNgXcI/

La Garganta Poderosa [@lagargantapoderosa]. (2020h, May 2). "A cada una de esas mujeres que están en los comedores comunitarios, les mando un abrazo caluroso y apretado. Ustedes son las que generan los verdaderos cambios en el mundo, las que están al frente de la pandemia luchando contra …" [Instagram photo]. Retrieved from https://www.instagram.com/p/COX8IMWg_Ai/

La Poderosa (2020a, April 25). Llegó el coronavirus a la villa 20. https://lapoderosa.org.ar/2020/04/llego-el-coronavirus-a-la-villa-20/

La Poderosa (2020b, May 7). 20 mil kilos de solidaridad. https://lapoderosa.org.ar/2020/05/20-mil-kilos-de-solidaridad/

Mazzini, C. & Ficoseco, V.S. (2020). Mujeres, militancias feminista y redes sociales. Análisis de la configuración de estereotipos en las páginas de medios de comunicación argentinos. *Question/Cuestión*, *2*(66), 1–38. URL: https://perio.unlp.edu.ar/ojs/index.php/question/article/view/6061/5410. DOI: 10.24215/16696581e485

Ortiz & Di Virgilio, M. (2020). Laboratorios de Vivienda (LAVs) Asentamientos precarios y vivienda social: Impactos del Covid-19-19 y respuestas. URL: https://www.uhph.org/sites/all/files/images/file/lav_Covid-19-19_lac_-_nota_conceptual_anexos_0.pdf

Oxfam (2020). El coronavirus no discrimina, las desigualdades sí: Vencer la pandemia requiere enfrentar las desigualdades. URL: https://oi-files-d8-prod.s3.eu-west-2.amazonaws.com/s3fs-public/2020-04/Covid-1919enLAC_notainformativa_.pdf

Pellecier, L. & Grasso, D. (2021, December 7). La pandemia dispara la desigualdad en todo el mundo. *Diario El País*, https://elpais.com/economia/2021-12-07/la-pandemia-dispara-la-desigualdad-en-todo-el-mundo.html

Pagani, G. & Gomez, Y. (2020). Emprendimientos con orientación social: Los casos de Hecho en Buenos Aires y La Garganta Poderosa. *HOLOGRAMATICA – Facultad de Ciencias Sociales*, *1*(33), 55–80 www.hologramatica.com.ar ISSN 1668-5024. URL: https://www.cienciared.com.ar/ra/usr/3/1922/holog33_v1_pp55_80.pdf

Porritelli, S. (2013). Palabras que rompen estigmas. https://www.centrocultural.coop/blogs/cooperativismo/2017/07/09/la-garganta-poderosa-palabras-que-rompen-estigmas

Rodo-Zárate, M. (2021). Metáforas, conceptos y aproximaciones sobre la interseccionalidad. Interseccionalidad. *Desigualdades, lugares y emociones*, 31–35. Bellaterra Edicions.

Scribano, A. (2012). Sociología del cuerpo/emoción. *RELACES. Revista Latinoamericana de Estudios sobre Cuerpos, Emociones y Sociedad*, *4*(10), 93–113. URL: http://www.relaces.com.ar/index.php/relaces/issue/view/6

Scribano, A. (2014). El don: Entre las prácticas intersticiales y el solidarismo. *Sociologias*, *16*(36), 74–103. Universidade Federal do Rio Grande do Sul Porto Alegre, Brasil. URL: https://seer.ufrgs.br/index.php/sociologias/article/view/49615/31026

Scribano, A. (2017a). *Normalization, enjoyment and bodies/emotions. Argentine sensibilities.* Nova Science Publishers.

Scribano, A. (2017b). Amor y acción colectiva: Una mirada desde las prácticas intersticiales en Argentina. *Aposta. Revista de Ciencias Sociales*, *74*, 241–280. URL: http://apostadigital.com/revistav3/hemeroteca/ascribano2.pdf

Scribano, A. (2020). *Love as a collective action: Latin America, emotions and interstitial practices.* Routledge.

Svampa, M. (2020). Reflexiones para un mundo post coronavirus. *NUSO*, abril. URL: https://nuso.org/articulo/reflexiones-para-un-mundo-post-coronavirus/

Testa, D. (2020). Quando o essencial se faz visível: Reflexões sobre a pandemia de Covid-1919 na Argentina. *Temáticas*, *28*(55), 301–313. DOI: 10.20396/tematicas.v28i55.14173

United Nations (2021, arch 25). The Covid-19 pandemic accelerates inequality and slows down Sustainable Development. URL: https://news.un.org/es/story/2021/03/1490032

Veiguela, N.Y., D'hers, V. (2021). Pandemia y nuevas redes. ¿La agroecología como escenario posible? [Conference Presentation] XIV Jornadas de Sociología, UBA. 1 to 5 November, Buenos Aires, Argentina.

6 Collective Action, Protest, and Covid-19 Restrictions: Offline and Online Community Participation in Italy and Australia

*Carlo Pistoni, Maura Pozzi, Emma F. Thomas,
and Craig McGarty*

Introduction

There are many different ways that people can seek to contribute to, or improve, the communities in which they live. Community participation can be enacted through engagement in civil society organisations and associations, which seek to bring about changes for people and their communities (Coplan et al., 2015). People can engage in their communities in different ways (e.g., social action, volunteerism, blood donation – see Pozzi et al., 2017), but the type that will receive most attention in this chapter is what is known as collective action. By collective action, we refer to a type of social activism in which people who identify themselves as a group in favour of a cause protest against an experienced or observed disadvantage (Mazzoni et al., 2015; Pozzi et al., 2017). These people can be called activists, defined as "people who actively work for social or political causes" (Curtin & McGarty, 2016, p. 228). All over the world, different associations organise collective actions and protests to fight for different issues, such as climate change and women's, LGBT+ people's, or workers' rights. Collective action has most commonly been understood as those actions of demonstration and protest that people act by taking to the streets, through signing petitions, demonstrations, or strikes (the so-called offline setting).

Contemporary social psychology has continued to emphasise the role of social identification in collective action (e.g., in the Social Identity Model of Collective Action, SIMCA, of van Zomeren et al., 2008; and the Encapsulation Model of Social Identity in Collective Action, EMSICA, of Thomas et al., 2012). That is, it is increasingly the case that collective action is understood as the expression of a shared sense of self by people who see themselves as acting together as part of a group. It follows that, during a time of acute upheaval to one's daily life, social relationships, and sense of self ("who I am" and "who we are"; identity), that collective action may also have been affected by the changes occasioned by the pandemic.

This chapter draws from the collective action literature to examine the process of mobilisation during the Covid-19 pandemic. This emergency

DOI: 10.4324/9781003301905-7

brought special attention to collective action, particularly because of public health restrictions. Indeed, most governments placed limits on gathering that inevitably limited the ways that people could express dissent: these included lockdown and physical distancing measures (measures that are often mislabelled as "social distancing"), travel bans, self-quarantines, and the stay-at-home orders have limited the ability of people to protest in traditional ways (offline), sometimes leaving online protests as the only option.

Different levels of social and economic restrictions were in place in different countries and in this chapter, we will look at the Italian and Australian experiences. The two contexts have experienced similar conditions, but in two different periods and modalities of restrictions. In Italy, since March 2020 the government applied very strong restrictive forms of preventive measures (i.e., the so-called lockdown), which, for several months, forbade people from leaving their homes, except for strictly essential reasons (e.g., going to purchase food). Up to the end of 2021, restrictive measures have continuously alternated, leading in other periods to total closures. In Australia, there were strong legal restrictions preventing protest across the nation in 2020 while in lockdown, and then again in areas under lockdown through 2021. Indeed, most of the population was locked down in the second half of 2021 and the virus spread rapidly in late 2021. So, in both contexts people had different opportunities to participate in collective actions by coming together and taking to the streets to protest.

In a context characterised by restrictions, social movements had to forcibly adapt their strategies of action and communication in order to continue to perform their tasks within the public sphere (Soler-i-Martí et al., 2020; Spear et al., 2020). This raises the question of how collective action took place in this emergency period and what impact those limits might have on people's future engagement. Though, Covid-19 has bridged the rapidly increasing use of internet and social media, leading new forms of technology to take a central role in social discussions. The use of online tools for collective action is not a new issue: next to the classic collective action (so-called offline collective action), there is a collective action that has moved online, which expresses itself through signing petitions online, liking or sharing content, or creating posts on social media (Lee et al., 2022). According to different authors (e.g., Lee et al., 2022; Xue & van Stekelenburg, 2018), online collective action can be defined as online activities promoted (and enacted) by Internet users aiming to settle a group disadvantage by influencing government policy decisions. Indeed, the pandemic has highlighted the importance of social media for people to find others with similar views and ideas and emotional reactions, coming to create a shared and group-based identification (Grant & Smith, 2021). Also, some scholars suggested that collective action, in its online form, has become easier, faster, and cheaper than in the offline form (e.g., Bennett et al. 2008): this could have an influence on people's participation in collective action, perhaps making it easier for people who have not usually engaged to participate and acting as a gateway to offline collective action (Velasquez & LaRose, 2015; Rohlinger & Bunnage, 2018;

but see Chayinska et al., 2021, for an alternative view). Given this context, we argue that the analysis of collective actions in this emergency context provides important insights into how civil society actors respond to restrictions.

In this chapter, using questionnaire data, we test two models of collective action and aim to explore how people who participate in civil society are engaged in online and offline collective action in Italy and Australia during the Covid-19 pandemic.

This chapter is organised into two sections. First, we present collective action literature, explaining the importance of studying its different forms in this specific historical context, where people's commitment has been limited by restrictions imposed by governments, acting on the advice of health authorities. Second, we explore how people engaged in collective action in Italy and Australia during the Covid-19 crisis, presenting results from the study. We conclude by highlighting results from the study and proposing reflections about how people have engaged in this specific historical context.

Collective Action in Offline and Online Settings

The main approaches that study collective action have shown that social identification is the strongest predictor of collective action and plays a central role in mobilisation (Stürmer & Simon, 2004; Thomas et al., 2012; van Zomeren et al., 2008). People who act to protest some state of affairs do so because they share a psychological sense of "who they are" with others who seek the same change. But where do such identities come from?

The current literature suggests that there are two distinct processes through which social identification may influence online and offline collective action, proposing two models: SIMCA by van Zomeren et al. (2008) and EMSICA by Thomas et al. (2012). Both models propose two complementary pathways to participation in collective action: 1) the "emotional" path, where people take action if/when they feel a relevant, action-oriented group-based emotion (Stürmer & Simon, 2009; Thomas et al., 2009; Wright & Lubensky, 2009), and 2) the "efficacy" path, where people take action if/when they believe that their group can achieve the goal of the collective action (van Zomeren et al., 2010; van Zomeren et al., 2004). Both models declare the central role of social identification but in different ways.

According to SIMCA, identification can have a direct effect on the intention to act but also an indirect effect through the mediation of the emotional and efficacy paths. Social identification can be considered the "conceptual and psychological bridge" (van Zomeren et al., 2008, p. 511) between the emotional and efficacy paths, producing these experiences: in SIMCA, emotions and efficacy derive from social identification with the group. This involves the existence of an already formed or pre-existing social identity that, through the mediation of other factors (feeling outraged about the situation and perceiving that they can achieve something as a group), leads people to act. Thus, people can be committed to other members of their national (e.g., Italian, Australian), occupational (e.g., health worker), community groups, or groups based on a specific opinion about how the world should be (e.g., Bliuc et al., 2007). These group memberships (social identities) then become the lens through which people perceive the world (including things that they think are unjust or outrageous) and assess whether or not group action can be effective (i.e., group efficacy; Bandura, 2000).

However, the authors of the SIMCA model stated that other causal ordering could be possible. Indeed, a model that explores a possible different causal explanation is EMSICA, in which the social identification mediates the effects of the emotions (i.e., capturing a sense of injustice) and efficacy beliefs, on the intention to participate in collective action. In EMSICA, emotion and efficacy causally precede social identification with the group. Rather, such identities emerge from this sense of indignation and efficacy about a specific situation. Thus, people may first perceive an unjust situation, believe that collective efforts can address it, and these reactions inform the commitment of novel or emergent groups. Literature shows how this process whereby social identification is central works for both offline and online collective action (Akfirat et al., 2021; Thomas et al., 2015).

In their original formulations, SIMCA and EMSICA did not address the role of morality in explaining why people act collectively. However, van Zomeren et al. (2012) explain that violated moral beliefs can fuel collective action against community disadvantage through their potentially strong normative fit to the content of a relevant social identification. A later extension by van Zomeren et al. (2012) shows that this third variable can also be considered in SIMCA as the "moral pathway", where moral beliefs about the actions performed are integrated, acting as an antecedent to the other two paths (see Figure 6.1). To date research has not yet considered the articulation of moral convictions in the context of the EMSICA. This chapter fills that gap to propose a possible integration of moral beliefs (see Figure 6.2). To better understand the effect of the models on online and offline engagement in

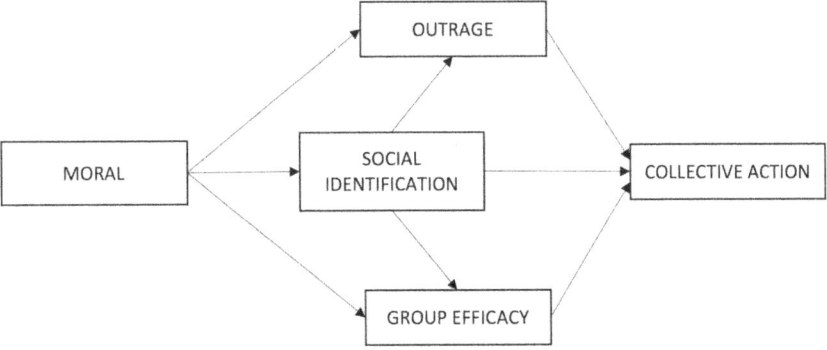

Figure 6.1 Extended social identity model of collective action (van Zomeren et al. 2012).

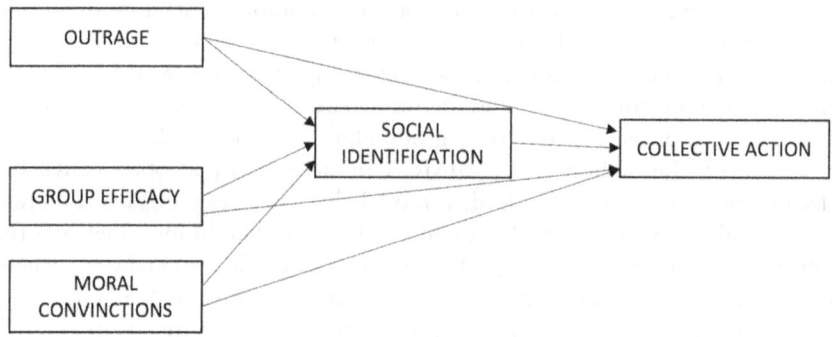

Figure 6.2 Proposed extended encapsulation model of social identity in collective action (adapted from Thomas et al. 2012).

collective action, we tested, for each nation, the Extended SIMCA and the proposed Extended EMSICA with two different outcomes: the first, future intentions to engage in offline collective action and the second, future intentions to engage in online collective action.

Returning to the pandemic context we discuss in this chapter, people seem to have experienced a strong sense of social identification with others (Ellena et al., 2021; Marzana et al., 2021), on the one hand, because of the shared situation with which they all had to cope, and on the other because they felt part of an extended group with shared goals of action (e.g., this was illustrated by people in Italy and other places who appeared on their balconies singing at certain times of the day or displaying signs or applauding health workers (e.g., La Repubblica, 2020a, 2020b). This sense of identification moved several solidarity actions and movements, which also led people to believe that "they could do it", increasing a sense of group efficacy (Jetten et al., 2020). In fact, it appears that the pandemic activated in people a shared sense of efficacy: the various actions proposed were also driven by a belief about the ability to succeed in having a possible concrete effect and that one's actions could have a real impact. Alongside this, actions were also characterised by feelings of anger and injustice, especially because of the pandemic and the resulting restrictions and governmental choices. Moreover, everything people felt seemed driven by the awareness that they were doing something they believed in and was right for them and the community at large (see Jetten et al., 2020).

Community Participation during the Covid-19 Crisis

To better understand how people engaged in efforts to improve the social and political standing of their communities during the Covid-19 pandemic, we conducted a survey in the context of online and offline collective action during the Covid-19 emergency context. A total of 157 participants were involved in

Italy and 620 participants in Australia, who were members of the broader community (i.e., not necessarily part of a specific movement or NGOs) who indicated that they participated in some form of social change action (e.g., signing petitions, public demonstrations). Participants were asked to complete a questionnaire[1] which measured the antecedents of engagement in collective action: social identification with other people that support the cause, outrage/anger (sense of injustice experienced by people due to social injustice), group efficacy (the sense of efficacy that people have in achieving a common goal), and moral convictions (moral beliefs about the actions). We also measured past behaviour and future intentions to engage in online and offline collective action (e.g., whether they had previously or intended to sign online and offline petitions, attend public demonstrations, write or share a post, take part in a strike).

To better capture the distinction between commitment to offline and online collective action, people's levels of engagement were compared. Specifically, we tested whether the means for past behaviour and future intention to behave differed for online and offline forms of collective action. In both Italy and Australia, participants reported greater intentions to engage in the future (both offline and online). Thus, people stated that they were more likely to act collectively in the future than they were in the past: this can be explained through the limitations imposed by governments on what social actions were possible. In fact, this may have both shaken people's desire to act but also made them realise how important engagement is to claim their rights, having experienced a context in which they could not manifest in the traditional way. Notably, however, people indicated greater intention to participate in online, relative to offline, collective actions in the future.

We then tested two extended classic models in the collective action literature: The Extended SIMCA (van Zomeren et al., 2012) and the new proposed Extended EMSICA (adapted from Thomas et al. 2012). It is important to point out that, based on the models shown above, for visual and explanatory clarity the model results will show only the significant paths.

Testing Extended SIMCA in Italy showed that social identification had a strong relation with both offline and online collective action and had a role of total mediator of moral convictions (Figure 6.3). Moreover, considering the intention to act collectively online, results showed that the efficacy path played a central role, acting as a partial mediator for intention to act. Results showed that the emotional pathway did not influence the intention to engage in offline and online collective action. Thus, our results did not support Extended SIMCA for the Italian sample. People seem to develop the intention to act collectively (both offline and online) thanks to the shared social identification based on the moral beliefs that they had regarding the topic of collective action. Moreover, regarding online collective action only, after moral beliefs had enabled identification with a social group, perceiving a sense of efficacy positively influenced the intention to act collectively online. However, social group identification did not lead to shared feelings of outrage in people's intention to act, either offline or online.

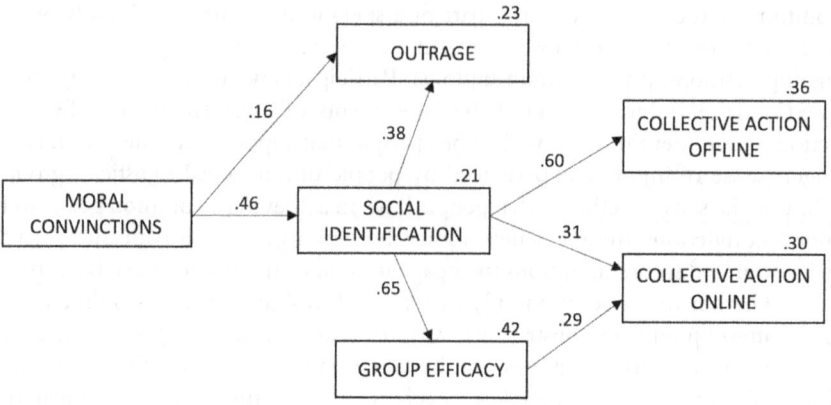

Figure 6.3 Extended SIMCA, Italian sample.

Note: Only significant paths are shown. Fit statistics: X2 = 13,280 df = 8 p = .103; CFI = .990; RMSEA = .065 CI:[.000; .125].

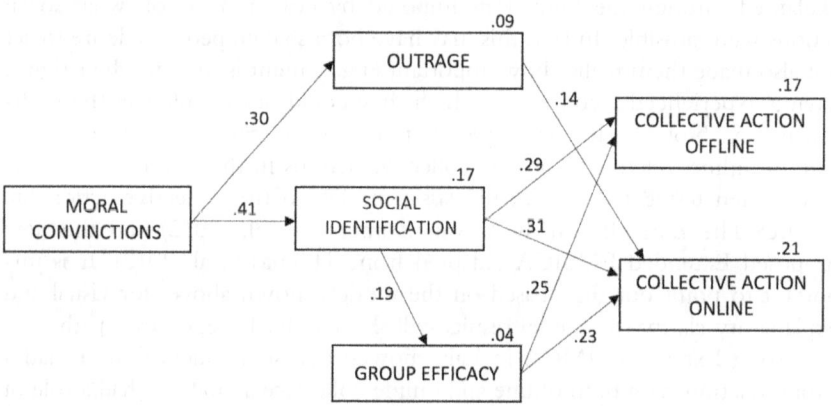

Figure 6.4 Extended SIMCA, Australian sample.

Note: Only significant paths are shown. Fit statistics: X2 = 33,296 df = 6 *p*<.001; CFI = .969; RMSEA = .086 CI:[.059; .115].

Testing Extended SIMCA in the Australian sample (Figure 6.4) showed that the moral and efficacy paths were the two paths that worked, indicating the central role of social identification as a total mediator between moral convictions and intention to act, while group efficacy was a partial mediator for intention to act, both offline and online. Moreover, considering intention to act collectively online, results show that all the paths played a central role: the emotional and identity paths were total mediators from the moral path to the intention to act online, while the efficacy path worked as in the offline model.

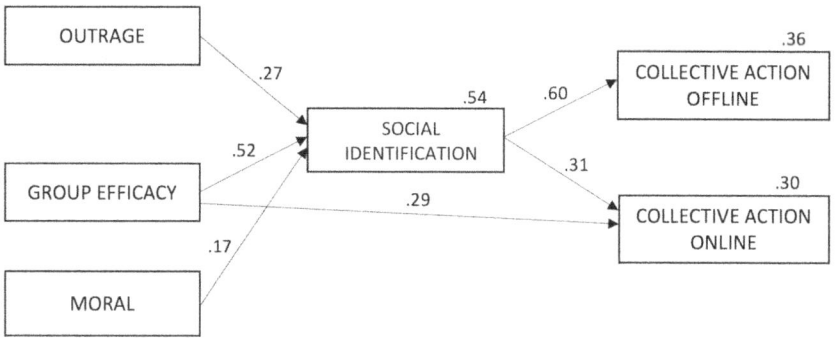

Figure 6.5 Extended EMSICA, Italian sample.

Note: Only significant paths are shown. Fit statistics: X^2 = 9,569 df = 5 p = .088; CFI = .985; RMSEA = .077 CI:[.000; .150].

Analysis also showed that the emotional pathway did not influence intention to engage in offline collective action. Thus, our results partially support Extended SIMCA. People develop the intention to act collectively offline by the creation of social identification based on the moral beliefs that people had regarding the topic of collective action, adding the central role of efficacy beliefs of achieving the aim of the collective action. While concerning the intention to act online, in addition to this, the process of the emotional path was added but separated from the other two. Indeed, strong moral convictions about the topic of the action positively influenced the experience of negative emotions about the topic itself, and this emotional activation positively influenced the intention to act collectively online.

Testing the Extended EMSICA (Figure 6.5) in Italy confirmed the importance of the three pathways in the emergence of social identification. In fact, unlike the proposed model (Figure 6.2), the emotional, efficacy, and moral pathways were totally mediated by social identification, in relation to offline action. Online action was similar except that social identification played a partial mediating role, also showing a direct relation between efficacy and action. Thus, the results provided greater support for the Extended EMSICA: it appears that people act both offline and online when their identification with the group becomes salient due to shared emotional activation, the belief that they can achieve their goal together, and via the presence of shared moral beliefs.

In Australia, the test of the Extended EMSICA (Figure 6.6) showed that regarding offline collective action, social identification was a partial mediator of the efficacy path, while a total mediator of the moral path. On the other hand, as far as online engagement is concerned, the model works the same, but with the addition of the emotional way, with only a direct relationship with the intention to act. However, the emotional path did not have an influence on the intention to act offline. Thus, results partially supported the Extended

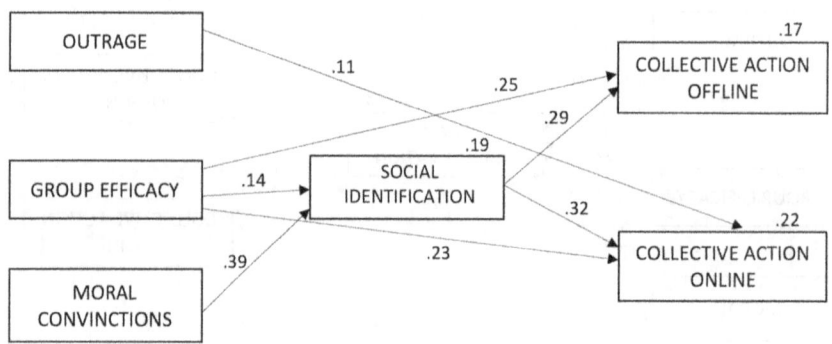

Figure 6.6 Extended EMSICA, Australian sample.

Note: Only significant paths are shown. Fit statistics: X2 = 2,505 df = 4 *p* = .644; CFI = 1.000; RMSEA = .000 CI:[.000; .049].

EMSICA. Regarding online collective action, in addition to forming identity through a sense of efficacy and shared moral beliefs (as for offline collective action), people's felt emotional responses to injustice also directly contributed to their intention to act.

Conclusions

The pandemic brought changes in every aspect of our lives but it also changed the nature of how we advocate for justice and equality within our local and national community. The results suggest that people were moved to express their desires about the world, particularly through online forms of collective action. Moreover, the findings underline the fundamental role of moral convictions: in these data, viewing one's cause in terms of fundamental right and wrong was consistently the precursor for allowing social identification to emerge. The fact of having moral convictions that motivate action is a good predictor of the formation of the sense of identity and, therefore, of the action itself. The data confirm the central role that people's identification with others plays, but especially in the causal order proposed by the EMSICA (Thomas et al., 2012). In both offline and online collective action, people experience feelings of collective outrage, efficacy, and moral conviction (as already argued), and it is these feelings that allow people to develop a commitment to others with whom they share a worldview (i.e., social identification). Because of this, people seem to seek out others with whom they can identify and create a shared vision of "who we are" and "what the community around us is": it is because of this shared vision that people take action, both offline and online.

Moreover, the data suggested that people were more likely to take collective action online than offline, perhaps explaining how the (forced) discovery of new modes of action may have made it easier for some people to engage, removing some of the barriers to participation that they may have confronted even before the pandemic (see Klandermans, 1997). People use the internet precisely as a means of finding other people with whom to share the same feelings (Akfirat et al., 2021). Perhaps collective action online has allowed people to find others similar to them in a simpler and, in a more immediate way, thus also facilitating an awareness that then leads to actual action. In addition, it has recently been pointed out that the EMSICA is a model that explains better than SIMCA why the general public may come to engage in collective action, especially in new and particular situations involving the broader community (Pozzi et al., 2022). This may lead us to hypothesise how the pandemic context (a specific situation that involved the broader community) may have affected the engagement of people who have not engaged in collective action in the past, leading them to develop feelings and a need to look for people who share those feelings, perhaps also through the use of the internet. The sense of efficacy plays a role in offline and online actions, thus leading people to identify and act because of a shared sense that they can achieve their goals by acting with other people. Moral conviction was found to be a new and interesting precursor to the intention to act collectively. Outrage and emotions related to collective action and social injustices turn out to be a key path to be investigated further and in more depth also in the general public (meaning people who have never protested in their lives – as shown in previous studies, see Pozzi et al., 2022) especially when online collective action can be exercised not necessarily by novel or emergent groups but also by "individual players". In fact, as already pointed out, online forms of engagement makes it easier even for individuals to act collectively (albeit on their own through their device).

We also observed evidence of intriguing cross-national variation in the data, however. Outrage seems to have played a different role in Italy, relative to Australia. On the one hand, in Italy the sense of outrage contributed to the emergence of the sense of identification (EMSICA) in both offline and online collective action (Figure 6.4). In Australia, on the other hand, in this sample and at this point in time, it seems that feeling outraged has a relationship only with online collective action: a direct relationship, where identification plays no role (Figure 6.6). This may suggest how certain online actions can also be driven at a more individual level (not going through social identification) by emotional activations, not going through other more "collective" feelings or considerations. In addition, the Italian and Australian samples were composed of activists and engaged people: perhaps outrage is not motivating these groups because instrumental concerns (e.g., efficacy) are more important. Moreover, as stated earlier, the pandemic has led people to perceive a shared sense of efficacy that their actions can have a concrete impact (Jetten et al., 2020); the potential implication of this is that a virtuous circle can occur in which people will increasingly participate in collective action, thanks precisely to this shared sense of efficacy.

Online collective action as a future way to engage seems to be a "simple" and immediate way to make one's voice heard, when people are unable to move around and when everyone's rights and liberties seem to be endangered, as the Covid-19 pandemic has shown (e.g., several people claimed, during the pandemic, that the ban on movement or gathering was a way of denying them their liberties and rights). Online forms of engagement can be an inclusive way of engaging people who cannot do so in the community and protests due, for example, to physical or health reasons.

In sum, as theorised by Meister (1969), depending on the type of participation an institution or association wants to promote (voluntary or provoked), it is important to know that in some situations, such as that related to a pandemic emergency, the emotional and cognitive pathways work differently. The first, the emotional path, has a strong impact especially in online forms of participation (see the Australian context). The second, the cognitive path, especially in group situations: it offers the possibility to show that one's own effectiveness, added to that of many others, allows to find "one's own in-group" with which to act. So, a protest that needs immediate and "quick" adherence could be more easily provoked by highlighting the emotional and outrage characters it might arouse. Certainly, creating a sense of belonging to a group and developing processes of identification with it appears to guarantee commitment to action for a cause, even during unprecedented barriers to such behaviours.

Note

1 This study was part of a larger study about collective behaviour and Covid-19 pandemic. Measures were non-specific and related to general situations of social injustice. Measures adapted from previous research were used: social identification (item example: "I feel I have many things in common with those people who participate in collective actions"; Thomas et al., 2012); outrage/anger (item example: "I feel outraged when I think of situations of social injustice"; Thomas et al., 2012); group efficacy (item example: "I think that those who participate in collective actions can achieve their goals"; Thomas et al., 2012); moral convictions (item example: "I feel that my position regarding social injustices is based on strong personal principles"; Hornsey et al., 2003).

References

Akfirat, S., Uysal, M.S., Bayrak, F., Ergiyen, T., Üzümçeker, E., Yurtbakan, T., & Özkan, Ö. S. (2021). Social identification and collective action participation in the internet age: A meta-analysis. *Cyberpsychology-Journal of Psychosocial Research on Cyberspace*, *15*(4). 10.5817/CP2021-4-10

Bandura, A. (2000). Exercise of human agency through collective efficacy. *Current Directions inPsychological Science*, *9*(3), 75–78. 10.1111/1467-8721.00064

Bennett, W.L., Breunig, C., & Givens, T. (2008). Communication and political mobilization: Digital media and the organization of anti-Iraq war demonstrations in the U.S. *Political Communication*, *25*(3), 269–289. 10.1080/10584600802197434

Bliuc, A.M., McGarty, C., Reynolds, K., & Muntele, D. (2007). Opinion-based group membership as a predictor of commitment to political action. *European Journal of Social Psychology*, *37*(1), 19–32. 10.1002/ejsp.334

Chayinska, M., Miranda, D., & González, R. (2021). A longitudinal study of the bidirectional causal relationships between online political participation and offline collective action. *Computers in Human Behavior, 121*, 106810. 10.1016/j.chb.2021.106810

Coplan, R.J., Ooi, L.L., & Rose-Klasnor, L. (2015). Naturalistic observations of schoolyard social participation: Marker variables for socio-emotional functioning in early adolescence. *The Journal of Early Adolescence, 35*(5-6), 628–650. 10.1177/0272431614523134

Curtin, N., & McGarty, C. (2016). Expanding on psychological theories of engagement to understand activism in context (s). *Journal of Social Issues, 72*(2), 227–241. 10.1111/josi.12164

Ellena, A.M., Aresi, G., Marta, E., & Pozzi, M. (2021). Post-traumatic growth dimensions differently mediate the relationship between national identity and interpersonal trust among young adults: A study on COVID-19 crisis in Italy. *Frontiers in Psychology, 11*. 10.3389/fpsyg.2020.576610

Grant, P.R., & Smith, H.J. (2021). Activism in the time of COVID-19. *Group Processes & Intergroup Relations, 24*(2), 297–305. 10.1177/1368430220985208

Hornsey, M.J., Majkut, L., Terry, D.J., & McKimmie, B.M. (2003). On being loud and proud: Non-conformity and counter-conformity to group norms. *British Journal of Social Psychology, 42*(3), 319–335. 10.1348/014466603322438189

Jetten, J., Reicher, S.D., Haslam, S.A., & Cruwys, T. (2020). *Together apart: The psychology of COVID-19.* Sage.

Klandermans, P.G. (1997). *The social psychology of protest.* Blackwell.

La Repubblica (2020a). *Coronavirus, balconi d'Italia in musica: il concerto che ha unito il Paese* [Coronavirus, balconies of Italy in music: the concert that united the country]. https://www.youtube.com/watch?v=7LbM8ZIP7pU

La Repubblica (2020b). *Coronavirus, Napoli: gli applausi spezzano il silenzio della città chiusa* [Coronavirus, Naples: applause breaks the silence of the closed city]. https://www.youtube.com/watch?v=11ZL_k6aDUI

Lee, Y., Tao, W., & Li, J.Y.Q. (2022). Motivations of online and offline activism against racism and xenophobia among Asian-American publics during the COVID-19 pandemic. *Telematics and Informatics, 67*, 101751. 10.1016/j.tele.2021.101751

Marzana, D., Novara, C., De Piccoli, N., Cardinali, P., Migliorini, L., Di Napoli, I., … & Procentese, F. (2021). Community dimensions and emotions in the era of COVID-19. *Journal of Community & Applied Social Psychology.* 10.1002/casp.2560

Mazzoni, D., Van Zomeren, M., & Cicognani, E. (2015). The motivating role of perceived right violation and efficacy beliefs in identification with the Italian water movement. *Political Psychology, 36*(3), 313–330. 10.1111/pops.12101

Meister, A. (1969). Participation, animation et dédeloppement à partir d'une étude rurale in Argentine. Paris: Édition Anthropos (trad. eng. Participation, associations, development, and change, Ross, New Brunswick, 1984).

Pozzi, M., Pistoni, C., & Alfieri, S. (2017). Verso una psicologia della partecipazione. Una sistematizzazione teorica dei rapporti tra le azioni nel sociale [Toward a Psychology of Participation: A theoretical analysis of the relationship between actions in the social context]. *Psicologia sociale, 12*(3), 253–276. 10.1482/87884

Pozzi, M., Passini, S., Chayinska, M., Morselli, D., Ellena, A.M., Włodarczyk, A., & Pistoni, C. (2022). 'Coming together to awaken our democracy': Examining precursors of emergent social identity and collective action among activists and non-activists in the 2019–2020 'Chile despertó' protests. *Journal of Community & Applied Social Psychology.* 10.1002/casp.2598

Rohlinger, D.A., & Bunnage, L.A. (2018). Collective identity in the digital age: Thin and thick identities in moveon.org and the tea party movement. *Mobilization*, *23*(2), 135–157. 10.17813/1086-671X-23-2-135

Soler-i-Martí, R., Ferrer Fons, M., & Terren, L. (2020). The interdependency of online and offline activism: A case study of Fridays For Future-Barcelona in the context of the COVID-19 lockdown. *Hipertext.net. 2020*, *21*, 105–114. 10.31009/hipertext.net.2020. i21.09

Spear, R., Erdi, G., Parker, M.A., & Anastasiadis, M. (2020) Innovations in Citizen Response to Crises: Volunteerism & Social Mobilization During COVID-19. *Interface: A Journal for and about Social Movements*, *12*(1), 1–9. https://halshs.archives-ouvertes.fr/ halshs-03027050

Stürmer, S., & Simon, B. (2004). Collective action: Towards a dual-pathway model. *European Review of Social Psychology*, *15*(1), 59–99. 10.1080/10463280340000117

Stürmer, S., & Simon, B. (2009). Pathways to collective protest: Calculation, identification, or emotion? A critical analysis of the role of group-based anger in social movement participation. *Journal of Social Issues*, *65*(4), 681–705. 10.1111/j.1540-4560.2009.01620.x

Thomas, E.F., McGarty, C., & Mavor, K.I. (2009). Aligning identities, emotions, and beliefs to create commitment to sustainable social and political action. *Personality and Social Psychology Review*, *13*(3), 194–218. 10.1177/1088868309341563

Thomas, E.F., McGarty, C., Stuart, A., Lala, G., Hall, L., & Goddard, A. (2015) Whatever happened to Kony2012? Understanding a global online phenomenon as an emergent social identity. *European Journal of Social Psychology*, *45*, 356–367. 10.1002/ejsp.2094

Thomas, F.E., Mavor, K., & McGarty, C. (2012). Social identities facilitate and encapsulate action-relevant constructs: A test of the social identity model of collective action. *Group Processes & Intergroup Relations*, *15*(1), 75–88. 10.1177/1368430211413619

van Zomeren, M., Leach, C.W., & Spears, R. (2010). Does group efficacy increase group identification? Resolving their paradoxical relationship. *Journal of Experimental Social Psychology*, *46*(6), 1055–1060. 10.1016/j.jesp.2010.05.006

van Zomeren, M., Postmes, T., & Spears, R. (2008). Toward an integrative social identity model of collective action: A quantitative research synthesis of three socio-psychological perspectives. *Psychological Bulletin*, *134*(4), 504–535. 10.1037/0033-2909.134.4.504

van Zomeren, M., Postmes, T., & Spears, R. (2012). On conviction's collective consequences: Integrating moral conviction with the social identity model of collective action. *British Journal of Social Psychology*, *51*(1), 52–71. 10.1111/j.2044-8309.2010.02000.x

van Zomeren, M., Spears, R., Fischer, A.H., & Leach, C.W. (2004). Put your money where your mouth is! Explaining collective action tendencies through group-based anger and group efficacy. *Journal of Personality and Social Psychology*, *87*(5), 649. 10.1037/ 0022-3514.87.5.649

Velasquez, A., & LaRose, R. (2015). Youth collective activism through social media: The role of collective efficacy. *New Media & Society*, *17*(6), 899–918. 10.1177/1461444813518391

Wright, S.C., & Lubensky, M.E. (2009). The struggle for social equality: Collective action versus prejudice reduction. In Demoulin, S., Leyens, J.-P., & Dovidio, J.F. (Eds.), *Intergroup misunderstandings: Impact of divergent social realities* (pp. 291–310). New York, NY: Psychology Press.

Xue, T., & van Stekelenburg, J. (2018). When the Internet meets collective action: The traditional and creative ways of political participation in China. *Current Sociology*, *66*(6), 911–928. 10.1177/0011392118783525

7 How can Covid Mutual Aid Groups be Sustained Over Time? The UK Experience

John Drury, Maria Fernandes-Jesus, Guanlan Mao, Evangelos Ntontis, Rotem Perach, and Daniel Miranda

Introduction

There was a sharp rise in informal social support activities in local communities in the UK during the Covid-19 pandemic in 2020–2021. One survey, in May 2020, found that 10 million people in the UK were involved in volunteering in response to the pandemic (Legal & General, 2020). Similarly, the World Happiness Report (Helliwell et al., 2022) noted that donations, volunteering, and helping strangers all showed increases in both 2020 and 2021. Also, the recent Kindness Test survey of over 60,000 people worldwide found that two thirds of respondents thought that the pandemic had made people kinder (Ingle, 2022). Yet a closer look at trends over time suggests a more complex picture, in which the initial rise in community support and general neighbourliness waned from the high point of Spring 2020 (Borkowska & Laurence, 2020; Lalot et al., 2021; Smith et al., 2020).

The trajectory of Covid mutual aid and similar community support groups in the UK can be seen as an expression of this overall rise and subsequent decline in informal support provision. In the first few weeks of March 2020, tens of thousands of people got involved in such groups (Booth, 2020), with over 4000 groups being set up in the first few months (Shabi, 2021). However, many Covid community support groups found it hard to sustain the morale and enthusiasm of volunteers[1] over time, and participation declined once "lockdown" restrictions started to ease (Tiratelli, 2020). For example, our analysis found that online activity in Covid-related Facebook mutual aid groups dropped by as much as 75% by June from the high point of March 2020 (Ntontis et al., 2022).

This pattern of public responses – a sharp increase in informal support behaviours, lasting a few months, and then a decline – is one commonly observed following disasters (Quarantelli, 1999).[2] However, needs for support remain strong even after the initial impact of the extreme event, and may continue long into the "recovery" period (Kaniasty & Norris, 1999). For example, 15 months after a large flooding incident in York, UK, Ntontis et al. (2020) found that for many residents of the flood-affected area, the community group and associated

DOI: 10.4324/9781003301905-8

support that was active in the early stages of the incident had long declined. Yet this period is precisely the time when those affected by flooding required practical and emotional support as they struggled with claiming insurance and rebuilding their homes (e.g., Mulchandani et al., 2019).

In the case of the Covid pandemic, from April 2020, the UK government provided a food delivery service, run by volunteers, for the most vulnerable (i.e., those shielding) (Gov.uk, 2021). The UK government also introduced a £500 self-isolation grant for those on low incomes, in September 2020. This was later enhanced by a discretionary fund plus a medicine delivery service (Reicher et al., 2021). However, £500 is less than the minimum wage, only about one in eight of the workforces were eligible (Reicher et al., 2021), and two thirds applying for self-isolation funds were turned down (Butcher & Cowling, 2021).

Therefore, in common with many other countries (Patel et al., 2021), the UK did not offer "wrap-around" support from the state for those having to self-isolate or shield. This meant that people relied on their family, friends, neighbours, or the wider community for help with many of their needs, especially shopping. Covid mutual aid and similar community support groups[3] responded to these needs, but also provided support in other ways to enable people to cope with the pandemic, including fundraising, providing information, dog-walking, mental health support, and collecting prescriptions (Curtin et al., 2021; Mao et al., 2021b). Not only this, but through their activities and new connections with their neighbours, many Covid mutual aid groups became aware of, and sought to respond to, other community needs beyond Covid, including among disadvantaged groups such as refugees and those suffering food poverty. Moreover, the first Covid wave and lockdown (in Spring 2020) was followed by further waves, again leading to high levels of self-isolation. Thus, as with other disasters, although the initial outpouring of support had declined following the first Covid wave, there were still many needs in the community not being met by the formal response. In other words, there was a continued need for mutual aid groups or similar support mechanisms.

Researching How Covid Mutual Aid Groups can be Sustained

The findings reported in this chapter are based on a programme of research that combined multiple methodologies, sources, and datasets to address the question of how Covid mutual aid groups can be sustained. First, a rapid review of existing research evidence, carried out in October 2020, enabled us to summarise existing knowledge on the broad area of public volunteering during the pandemic (Mao et al., 2021b). Second, to establish with primary data not only the rise but also the decline of mutual aid group activity that commenters had noted (e.g., Tiratelli, 2020), we analysed social media activity in a large sample of UK mutual aid groups (Ntontis et al., 2022). This analysis established that requests for support declined in a similar way to offers of support and that there was only minimal evidence of an uptick when the second pandemic wave occurred in Autumn 2020. Next, to explore the experiences of Covid mutual aid group participants, and in particular the extent to which participation could provide wellbeing benefits, we carried out an interview study with 11 volunteers in a mutual aid group organised by ACORN, a community union and anti-poverty campaigning organisation (Mao et al., 2021a). To understand Covid mutual aid group organisers' perspectives on the factors that helped sustain their groups, we interviewed 32 of them from different parts of the UK about the resources and support they needed, their strategies for retaining volunteers, and some of the experiences they felt motivated people to continue to participate (Fernandes-Jesus et al., 2021). Finally, we carried out a two-wave questionnaire survey of 600 mutual aid participants to test the links between the various strategies, experiences, and continued involvement.

The question of how Covid mutual aid groups can be sustained over time is not simply one for academic research, as it is a profoundly practical question. Rather than focusing on cognitive predictors of participation (as is common in research on collective action), we were principally concerned with the actions of groups and their organisers to consciously create the conditions for those "predictors" – that is, we focus on organisers' conscious *strategies* (cf. Tekin & Drury, 2021). Our programme of research was therefore more than just data-gathering by academics coming from the outside. It aimed to be participatory and to have impact by assisting mutual aid groups in the Covid response. The research designs and analysis were based on collaboration with an advisory group of Covid mutual aid group organisers; and findings have been shared and discussed in dialogue events with Covid mutual aid group participants and others in the voluntary sector where there has been common learning on "what works" in sustaining mutual aid groups over time.

We summarise the research findings in three sections. First, an obvious starting point for sustaining mutual aid groups is material support – or *scaffolding* – for those groups. Second, we consider how volunteers *experience* participating in the group, and finally we discuss what the organisers can do to *facilitate that (positive) group experience* (and mitigate negative experiences).

Group Scaffolding

Participants in UK Covid mutual aid and other Covid community support groups were motivated by many of the psychological factors that have been found to predict participation in volunteering and collective action, including community identification (Tekin et al., 2021; Wakefield et al., 2022), identification with the role of volunteer (Wakefield et al., 2022), allyship (Tekin et al., 2021), compassion for local people (Abrams et al., 2020), sense of community responsibility (Toubøl et al., 2022), and sense of injustice (Mao et al., 2021a).

However, while many people in the community might have these motivations, not everyone will be able to act upon them. Covid mutual aid group organisers we spoke to stressed that the fundamental basis of a group able to provide support to others during the pandemic was the material and practical support the group itself received (Fernandes-Jesus et al., 2021). Thus, the coordinators we spoke to emphasised the need for donations (both financial and food), resources such as transport loaned to them from other organisations, computing facilities and equipment, and meeting and storage locations.

Relationships with other organisations were often crucial to getting these material resources (Fernandes-Jesus et al., 2021). Mutual aid groups were often not in a position to apply for grant funding directly, for example, and relied on their relationship with registered charities and other organisations who were able to do so. Similarly, local authorities were able to help Covid mutual aid groups with funding and with space; and in some cases but not others this support was indeed provided. Organisers saw relationships of trust both with the local community and with other organisations as fundamental (Fernandes-Jesus et al., 2021). In line with this point, our survey of participants found that the alliances their group had with other groups were a significant predictor of intentions to participate in the future, particularly for those participants with little previous community participation experience.

Discussion of scaffolding and relationships with other organisations highlighted some tensions as well as needs among Covid mutual aid groups. Some organisers suggested that people in their role should receive a salary: *"I think it's more sustainable for the organisation to have a full-time employee with that as their job, they're paid for it, and they can look over, they can monitor what's going on in the organisation"*. (Interviewee, East Dunbartonshire). In addition, some groups discussed registering as charities (in order to apply for grants) or other forms of professionalisation and formal organisation. Yet such developments threatened their identity as independent and the "grassroots" nature of their organisation that was the key to their good relationship with local people (Fernandes-Jesus et al., 2021; Mao et al., 2021a).

Coordinators also referred to volunteers as a basic resource too, and highlighted the need for volunteers with particular skills such as experience in public health and social services; experience in community organising and project management; IT and digital skills; leadership and communication skills (Fernandes-Jesus, 2021). Attracting and retaining such volunteers was a function of those participants having continued motivations or positive experiences from being in the group.

Group Experiences

Our interviews with participants indicated that volunteering in mutual aid groups could be stressful and distressing at times (Mao et al., 2021a). Volunteers reported discomfort when witnessing the difficult life situations of those they were helping. Going to the homes of those who were isolated, disadvantaged or suffering from racism, among participants who often came from a more middle-class background, created a feeling of intruding and being part of the privileged group. In addition, the risk of spreading infection – both to self and to vulnerable people – created stress for volunteers, who were aware that a mistake could be life-threatening. In addition, the organisers we interviewed reported that the activity could be extremely tiring and that there was a risk of burnout (Fernandes-Jesus et al., 2021).

Yet participating in Covid mutual aid groups is also associated with well-being (Bowe et al., 2021). Our interviews with volunteers explored a number of sources and mechanisms of such wellbeing (Mao et al., 2021a). First, interviewees reported that by participating in the Covid mutual aid group they felt good about themselves – they were "making a difference", helping others, and acting in line with their values. Having such an impact felt emotionally positive. Some participants also reported an increased sense of engagement with life, suggesting that the mental health benefits of participating in the mutual aid group positively affected other areas of their life. These good feelings were reinforced by the positive feedback they received from the people they helped.

Bowe et al.'s (2021) survey of over 200 Covid community support participants suggests that two potential mechanisms of enhanced wellbeing are a greater sense of community identification and unity. In other words, participating in Covid community support groups could transform relationships and hence the sense of self based on those relationships. In our interviews with volunteers (Mao et al., 2021a), some described new relationships with other volunteers and with the recipients of support. A new sense of camaraderie or shared group membership with a wider group of people provided them with expectations of social support. In line with Bowe et al.'s survey, some also described a greater sense of connection to their local community, a finding repeated in our interviews with coordinators (Fernandes-Jesus et al., 2021).

These new forms of social identification matter for wellbeing, since shared social identity is associated not only with expectations of social support – as above – but also with efficacy and related experiences (subjective control, empowerment), all of which themselves predict wellbeing (Drury et al., 2015; Ntontis et al., 2021). Thus, some of our interviewees were explicit that participating in the mutual aid group made them feel less helpless, and gave them a greater sense of agency. In some cases, the activity created a sense of confidence and collective empowerment – including the capacity to challenge the injustices they witnessed (Mao et al., 2021a).

Our interviews with organisers similarly referred to experiences of efficacy as well as the development of new skills – including practical knowledge of community organising, how to deal with people in group settings, how to assume leadership roles, communication skills, and how to listen to people's needs (Fernandes-Jesus et al., 2021). These experiences were in turn associated with positive emotions of pride and joy as well as wellbeing.

The wellbeing benefits evidenced in our interviews with volunteers were not evenly spread. Looking closely at the different backgrounds and expectations of the participants, there appeared to be differences according to the extent to which participants came to the Covid mutual aid group as activists or not (Mao et al., 2021a). Those volunteers with a relatively apolitical identity were more likely to report a new connectedness or camaraderie. By contrast, those with a politicised collective identity (Simon & Klandermans, 2001) were more likely to express feelings of empowerment as a result of this identity: being in the group enabled them to realise their (political) values. Among these interviewees, their political values were realised in three main ways. First, participating in the group was a way to reclaim agency since the activity served to create a solution to what they perceived as the government's inadequate response to Covid. Second, participation not only contributed to the Covid response, it was also a way to grow the community union ACORN and therefore challenge those in power more effectively in the future. Third, for participants the effectiveness of the mutual aid group contrasted with the "transactional" (and ineffective) practices of existing society and therefore served as a kind of validation of their beliefs in the principles of mutual aid.

Facilitating Group Experiences

For those organising Covid mutual aid groups, the task they face is not only "external" (in this case supporting the community) but also "internal" (sustaining the group in order to support the community). Here we summarise our findings on organisers' strategies to maintain volunteer participation (Fernandes-Jesus et al., 2021) – by trying to protect volunteers from negative experiences and to enhance the experiences thought to motivate continued involvement.

In several of their stated strategies, one aim of organisers was to enhance participants' sense of belonging in and identification with the Covid mutual aid group (cf. Wakefield et al., 2022), and several of them stated that their volunteers did indeed feel part of the group. One of the ways to achieve this responded to the stressors we mentioned earlier. Organisers talked about creating a culture of care and support. They developed guidelines to reduce risk of infection and they monitored workloads to ensure that volunteers were not overloaded. Similarly, our rapid review (Mao et al., 2021b) found that among the factors identified by groups as being important for successful retention of volunteers was not asking volunteers to engage in activities they were uncomfortable with (McCabe et al., 2020).

As part of this culture of care and support, most organisers we spoke to emphasised the role of regular communication within the group. Such communication involved not only informing volunteers, but also listening to their needs. Some of the groups held meetings specifically to share experiences and understand each other's needs.

Meetings and events where people in the Covid mutual aid group could socialise was another important way of getting volunteers to feel part of the group and thereby sustain their participation (cf. Ntontis et al., 2020). Where in-person meetings were not possible, groups organised online meetings.

Organisers said that the structure of the group was important in making people feel part of it and motivating continued involvement. While there was typically a division between those who played an organising role and other participants (i.e., volunteers, many of whom would come and go), organisers referred to implementing "horizontal" organisation (cf. Chevée, 2021) and shared informal leadership as a way of building a sense of inclusion. Thus, some organisers described the way their groups made decisions collectively, rather than a minority making all the decisions.

Our two-wave survey of volunteers was an opportunity to examine the effectiveness of some of the strategies described by organisers. We found that perceptions of a culture of group care were associated with later reports that there was good communication in the group, though good communication was not found to be a predictor of continued participation. Perceptions of a culture of care in the group also predicted subsequent sense of community responsibility; and sense of community responsibility predicted both subsequent well-being and intentions to participate in the future. Feeling supported by the group and sense of community responsibility predicted subsequent identification with the local community, which has been found by other research to be a predictor of Covid support group participation (Tekin et al., 2021; Wakefield et al., 2022).

The survey also found some differences between volunteers with previous experience of community participation or political activism and those without, which is likely to be important for those organisers trying to keep participants engaged. Thus, for those with previous community participation experience (but not other participants), attending socialising events predicted subsequent intentions to participate in the Covid mutual aid group and beyond. In addition, for those with previous community participation experience, their identification with the Covid mutual aid group was a predictor of subsequent amount of participation reported. For those with little experience of political activism, sense of community responsibility predicted both subsequent reported amount of participation and future intentions. By contrast, for those with previous experience of political activism, good communication in the group was a predictor of subsequent intentions of future participation.

Prospects for UK Mutual Aid Groups

Two years after the start of the first "lockdown", the UK government dropped almost all measures designed to counter the Covid pandemic, including the legal requirement to self-isolate, relying just on the vaccination programme. In addition, very likely the increased availability of supermarket delivery slots solved the problem of shopping for most of those who were self-isolating. Mutual aid groups are now much less active and visible than in the early days of the pandemic. So does the question of how to sustain these groups still matter?

We would argue that sustaining the mutual aid groups that arose in the pandemic remains important, for a number of reasons. Many of the organisers we spoke to wanted to continue to respond to community needs beyond

Covid (Fernandes-Jesus et al., 2021). Those groups that continued after the early waves of the pandemic extended their activities to other purposes in their local community, including sharing food, pooling DIY tools, measures to tackle unscrupulous landlords, managing a community garden (Shabi, 2021), and tackling homelessness (Lang, 2021). First, then, Covid (or even post-Covid) mutual aid groups are still responding to community needs, and in order to do that the groups themselves need to be maintained.

Second, the mutual aid groups that are still active face new challenges. Some have taken the decision to apply for charitable status so that they get access to funding (Power & Benton, 2021). Many others continue with their more informal status. Mutual aid groups cannot replace public services and it should be clear that the needs they are meeting represent a failure of the social safety-net the state should provide. Nevertheless, such groups do have a role complementing the work of local authorities, charities, and local infrastructure organisations. These organisations should develop relationships with mutual aid groups to support their activities (with expertise, funds, and connections) – so long as this is in a way that does not undermine the groups' identity and appeal as informal, grassroots, and independent (Power & Benton, 2021).

Relatedly, where Covid mutual aid groups have disbanded and formal volunteer organisations and local infrastructure organisations have stepped in to meet the residual local needs, there may be a new reservoir of people inspired by their experience of involvement in mutual aid groups – and who through the experience now identify as "volunteers" or "community activists" (Bowe et al., 2021) – who will need to be coordinated and offered volunteering opportunities (Scottish Government, 2022). Certainly, the mutual aid movement changed the volunteer demographic and introduced many new people to community activity (Mao et al., 2021b).

Finally, while the worst of the Covid pandemic may be over in the UK, at the time of writing (May 2022), Covid infection rates are still very high as are numbers of hospitalisations and deaths. The pandemic is not over, despite the UK government's messaging and the disappearance of Covid from the headlines. There are still people in need; and with the likelihood of new variants, there will continue to be needs for support in the foreseeable future.

Recommendations

Our programme of research on and dialogue with Covid mutual aid groups suggests a number of recommendations for organisers seeking to sustain their groups and retain volunteers over time. First, groups need practical resources such as storage space, transport, and computing facilities. A salary for organisers would help many groups, but this and other financial support should come without interference in the group's autonomy and flexibility. As mutual aid groups often rely on other organisations, helping them to create new connections and relationships is important for sustaining them.

Second, as well as practical needs there are the psychological aspects. Organisers are often already employing the effective strategies we identified in the research. But becoming more aware of "what works" and for who, and how it links to positive experiences in volunteers, will help organisers use their strategies more effectively. The most important strategies in our findings included building shared identities with volunteers; promoting a culture of group care; providing socialising events and meetings; open communication; and flexible or horizontal organisation.

Mutual aid groups were crucial in the response to Covid-19 in 2020 (Kaye & Tiratelli, 2020). While they were relatively novel in the UK in the Covid-19 pandemic, community participation more broadly is well known to be vital in strategies to combat disease outbreaks (Costello, 2020). Understanding how to support and sustain (Covid) mutual aid and similar groups will be a vital part of emergency response in the next crisis.

Acknowledgements

The authors thank all participants for sharing their experiences and time. The research described in this chapter was supported by funding from the Economic and Social Research Council to John Drury and Evangelos Ntontis (grant reference ES/V005383/1). We thank Sanj Choudhury for assistance in preparing the manuscript.

Notes

1 The word "volunteer" can mean quite different things within the context of mutual aid. Some groups resist the term as it implies a relationship of charity rather than solidarity. For other groups, however, it captures the fact that some participants see themselves as different from the group organisers. In this chapter, for convenience, we will use the term "volunteer" interchangeably with "group member".
2 The Covid pandemic can be considered a kind of disaster, despite being more dispersed in time and space than earthquakes, fires and so on, as here too there has been a collective threat of death and a requirement for urgent response.
3 While a large number of groups called themselves "mutual aid" and looked to that tradition of organising for their principles, others were already existing community support groups that re-purposed, or new informal groups that didn't call themselves "mutual aid" (Mao et al., 2021b).

References

Abrams, D., Lalot, F., Broadwood, J., & Platts-Dunn, I. (2020, July). *Beyond us and them: Perception of Covid-19 and social cohesion*. Belong – The Cohesion and Integration Network. https://www.belongnetwork.co.uk/resource-centre/resources/beyond-us-and-them-perception-of-Covid-19-and-social-cohesion-july-2020-report/.

Booth, R. (2020, March 20). Community aid groups set up across UK amid coronavirus crisis. *The Guardian.* https://www.theguardian.com/society/2020/mar/16/community-aid-groups-set-up-across-uk-amid-coronavirus-crisis

Borkowska, M., & Laurence, J. (2020). Coming together or coming apart? Changes in social cohesion during the Covid-19 pandemic in England. *European Societies, 23*(1), 1–19. https://www.tandfonline.com/doi/full/10.1080/14616696.2020.1833067

Bowe, M., Wakefield, J., Kellezi, B., Stevenson, C., McNamara, N., Jones, B., Sumich, A., & Heym, N. (2021). The mental health benefits of community helping during crisis: Coordinated helping, community identification and sense of unity during the Covid-19 pandemic. *Journal of Community and Applied Social Psychology, 32*(3), 521–535. 10.1002/casp.2520

Butcher, B., & Cowling, P. (2021). Covid: How many people get self-isolation payments? *BBC.* https://www.bbc.co.uk/news/56201754

Chevée, A. (2021). Mutual aid in North London during the Covid-19 pandemic. *Social Movement Studies, 21*(4), 413–419. 10.1080/14742837.2021.1890574

Costello, A. (2020). *A social vaccine for Ebola. A lesson for the Democratic Republic of Congo.* https://www.anthonycostello.net/2018/05/20/a-social-vaccine-for-ebola-a-lesson-for-the-democratic-republic-of-congo

Curtin, M., Rendall, J.S., Roy, M.J., & Teasdale, S. (2021). *Solidarity in a time of crisis: The role of mutual aid to the Covidovid-19 pandemic.* Yunus Centre for Social Business and Health/Glasgow Caledonian University. https://www.cso.scot.nhs.uk/wp-content/uploads/COVCGU2006.pdf

Drury, J., Evripidou, A., & Van Zomeren, M. (2015). Empowerment: The intersection of identity and power in collective action. In D. Sindic, M. Barreto, & R. Costa-Lopes (Eds.), *Power and identity* (pp. 94–116). London: Psychology Press.

Fernandes-Jesus, M., Mao, G., Ntontis, E., Cocking, C., McTague, M., Schwarz, A., Semlyen, J., & Drury, J. (2021). More than a Covid-19 response: Sustaining mutual aid groups during and beyond the pandemic. *Frontiers in Psychology, 12,* 1–17. 10.3389/fpsyg.2021.716202

Gov.uk. (2021). Coronavirus (Covid-19): Accessing food and essential supplies.United Kingdom Department for Environment, Food & Rural Affairs. https://www.gov.uk/guidance/coronavirus-Covid-19-accessing-food-and-essential-supplies#if-youre-having-difficulty-shopping

Helliwell, J.F., Layard, R., Sachs, J.D., De Neve, J-E., Aknin, L.B., & Wang, S. (Eds.). (2022). *World Happiness Report 2022.* New York: Sustainable Development Solutions Network. https://worldhappiness.report/

Ingle, A. (2022, March 9). *Two thirds of people who took part in The Kindness Test think the pandemic has made people kinder.* University of Sussex. https://www.sussex.ac.uk/news/article/57570-two-thirds-of-people-who-took-part-in-the-kindness-test-think-the-pandemic-has-made-people-kinder

Kaniasty, K., & Norris, F. (1999). The experience of disaster: Individuals and communities sharing trauma. In R. Gist & B. Lubin (Eds.), *Response to disaster: Psychosocial, community, and ecological approaches* (pp. 25–62). Bruner/Mazel.

Kaye, S., & Tiratelli, L. (2020, July 13). Communities vs coronavirus: The rise of mutual aid. *New Local.* https://www.newlocal.org.uk/publications/communities-vs-coronavirus-the-rise-of-mutual-aid/

Lalot, F., Abrams, D., Broadwood, J., Davies Hayon, J., & Platts-Dunn, I. (2021). The social cohesion investment: Communities that invested in integration programmes are showing greater social cohesion in the midst of the Covid-19 pandemic. *Journal of Community and Applied Social Psychology, 32*(3), 536–554. 10.1002/casp.2522

Lang, M.J. (2021, December 30). *Mutual aid groups formed amid the pandemic have turned their focus to the homeless. The Washington Post.* https://www.washingtonpost.com/dc-md-va/2021/12/30/mutual-aid-homeless-response/

Legal & General (2020). Press release: 10 million Brits volunteering as the nation unites in the Isolation Economy, says Legal & General. https://group.legalandgeneral.com/en/newsroom/press-releases/10-million-brits-volunteering-as-the-nation-unites-in-the-isolation-economy-says-legal-general

Mao, G., Drury, J., Fernandes-Jesus, M., & Ntontis, E. (2021a). How participation in Covid-19 mutual aid groups affects subjective wellbeing and how political identity moderates these effects. *Analyses of Social Issues and Public Policy, 21*(1), 1082–1112. 10.1111/asap.12275

Mao, G., Fernandes-Jesus, M., Ntontis, E., & Drury, J. (2021b). What have we learned so far about Covid-19 volunteering in the UK? A rapid review of the literature. *BMC Public Health, 21,* 1470. 10.1186/s12889-021-11390-8

McCabe, A., Wilson, M., & Paine, A.E. (2020, October 13). Stepping up and helping out: Grassroots volunteering in response to Covid-19. *Local Trust.* https://localtrust.org.uk/insights/research/briefing-6-rapid-research-Covid-19/

Mulchandani, R., Smith, M., Armstrong, B., English National Study of Flooding and Health Study Group, Beck, C.R., & Oliver, I. (2019). Effect of insurance-related factors on the association between flooding and mental health outcomes. *International Journal of Environmental Research and Public Health, 16*(7), 1174.

Ntontis, E., Drury, J., Amlôt, R., Rubin, G.R., & Williams, R. (2020). Endurance or decline of emergent groups following a flood disaster: Implications for community resilience. *International Journal of Disaster Risk Reduction, 45,* 1–29. 10.1016/j.ijdrr.2020.101493

Ntontis, E., Drury, J., Amlôt, R., Rubin, J.G., Williams, R., & Saavedra, P. (2021). Collective resilience in the disaster recovery period: Emergent social identity and observed social support are associated with collective efficacy, wellbeing, and the provision of social support. *British Journal of Social Psychology, 60,* 1075–1095. 10.1111/bjso.12434

Ntontis, E., Fernandes-Jesus, M., Mao, G., Dines, T., Kane, J., Karakaya, J., Perach, R., Cocking, C., McTague, M., Schwartz, A., Semlyen, J., & Drury, J. (2022). Tracking the nature and trajectory of social support in Facebook mutual aid groups during the Covid-19 pandemic. *International Journal of Disaster Risk Reduction, 76,* 1–15. 10.1016/j.ijdrr.2022.103043

Patel, J., Fernandes, G., & Sridhar, D. (2021). How can we improve self-isolation and quarantine for Covid-19?. *BMJ, 372,* 1–6. https://www.bmj.com/content/372/bmj.n625

Power, A., & Benton, E. (2021, May 6). Where next for Britain's 4,300 mutual aid groups? *LSE.* https://blogs.lse.ac.uk/Covid19/2021/05/06/where-next-for-britains-4300 mutual-aid-groups/

Quarantelli, E.L. (1999). *Disaster related social behavior: Summary of 50 years of research findings.* University of Delaware Disaster Research Center. http://dspace.udel.edu/handle/19716/289

Reicher, S., Drury, J., & Michie, S. (2021). Contrasting figures on adherence to self-isolation show that support is even more important than ever. *BMJ Opinion.* https://blogs.bmj.com/bmj/2021/04/05/why-contrasting-figures-on-adherence-to-self-isolation-show-that-support-to-self-isolate-is-even-more-important-than-we-previously-realised/

Scottish Government. (2022, January 31). *Coronavirus (Covid-19) volunteering – third sector perspectives: Survey report.* Scottish Government. https://www.gov.scot/publications/scottish-third-sector-perspectives-volunteering-during-Covid-19-survey-report/pages/11/

Shabi, R. (2021, September 8). Stronger communities are emerging out of the wreckage of the pandemic. *The Guardian.* https://www.theguardian.com/commentisfree/2021/sep/08/pandemic-mutual-aid-politics-food-banks-welfare-state

Simon, B., & Klandermans, B. (2001). Politicized collective identity: A social psychological analysis. *American Psychologist, 56*(4), 319–331.

Smith, L.E., Duffy, B., Moxham-Hall, V., Strang, L., Wessely, S., & Rubin, G.J. (2020). Anger and confrontation during the Covid-19 pandemic: A national cross-sectional survey in the UK. *Journal of the Royal Society of Medicine, 114*(2), 77–90, 0141076820962068. https://journals.sagepub.com/doi/full/10.1177/0141076820962068

Tekin, S., & Drury, J. (2021). Silent Walk as a street mobilization: Campaigning following the Grenfell Tower fire. *Journal of Community and Applied Social Psychology, 31*(4), 425–437. 10.1002/casp.2521

Tekin, S., Sager, M., Bushey, A., Deng, Y., & Uluğ, Ö. M. (2021). How do people support each other in emergencies? A qualitative exploration of altruistic and prosocial behaviours during the Covid-19 pandemic. *Analyses of Social Issues and Public Policy, 21*(1), 1113–1140. 10.1111/asap.12277

Tiratelli, L. (2020, October 1). A second wave for mutual aid? *New Local.* https://www.newlocal.org.uk/articles/a-second-wave-for-mutual-aid/

Toubøl, J., Carlsen, H.B., Nielsen, M.H., & Brincker, B. (2022). Mobilizing to take responsibility: Exploring the relationship between Sense of Community Responsibility (SOC-R), Public Service Motivation (PSM) and public service resilience during Covid-19. *Public Management Review.* 10.1080/14719037.2021.2018847

Wakefield, H., Bowe, M., & Kellezi, B. (2022). Who helps and why? A longitudinal exploration of volunteer role identity, between-group closeness, and community identification as predictors of coordinated helping during the Covid-19 pandemic. *British Journal of Social Psychology, 61*(3), 907–923. 10.1111/bjso.12523

Appendix: Resources

Our project website brings together a range resources for (Covid) mutual aid groups, including examples of community solidarity from five different Covid mutual aid groups; lessons from activists and social movements pre-Covid; our mutual aid toolbox of tips compiled from the experiences of the organisers we spoke to; and a large collection of articles on Covid mutual aid groups in the UK and beyond: https://www.sussex.ac.uk/research/projects/groups-and-Covid/community-support-and-mutual-aid

Part II

Communities Transforming Social Representations and Public Policies

8 Reimagining Infrastructure of Care in the Pandemic Time: Sketches from Kolkata

Raktim Ray, Amit Chatterjee, Koumi Dutta, and Dana Sousa Limbu

Introduction

"We, some students at Presidency University, usually donate some money to feed the street children in College Street Kolkata. We usually keep the money with the security guard of our university. When the lockdown started, we could not go to the university and hand over the money to the guards. One day, one of the security guards called me and mentioned that the street children were suffering from acute hunger as the guards could not provide money for buying them some food. After hearing this, I connected with my friends who were also thinking as news of acute hunger kept reaching our ears. Finally, we managed to get a private vehicle to commute to College Street and bought some foods for the street children. We also realised that the lockdown would be prolonged by that time, and we needed to do something to feed these children. We thought of running a small community kitchen with the money we had. That is how the idea of a solidarity network came into the picture".

(Koumi)

This reflection from Koumi was not a unique story of crisis during the pandemic in India. First, the pandemic has exposed the vulnerability and temporariness of urban living at the margins by continuous ruptures through uncertainty. Second, the socio–spatial materiality of infrastructure was changed due to reduced mobility (because of lockdowns) and social distancing. We position our chapter at this juncture and explore how the absence of certain infrastructures and inadequacy of the state support provided new forms of infrastructure through "networked mobilisation" of social capital. In this chapter, we also formulate solidarity networks as a form of infrastructure which provided care to the people at the urban margins. Drawing on data from our ethnographic fieldwork with such a solidarity network Quarantined Student-Youth Network (QSYN) from Kolkata, this chapter provides an alternative framework to understand how politics of care is operationalised through solidarity networks and locates care at the centre of theorisation of the infrastructure in the postcolonial urban context. By doing so, it not only helps

DOI: 10.4324/9781003301905-10

us to reformulate the normative discourse around infrastructure but also argues for a contextual and generative theorisation of the postcolonial urban context.

After the introductory discussion, the chapter critically engages with the work on politics of care and solidarity networks in its second section. The section then connects it with the literature focusing on care during the pandemic. This section also discusses the popular imagination around urban infrastructures and adopts the framework of "people as infrastructure" (Simone, 2004) to establish this chapter's arguments. The third section of this chapter contextualises the study in Kolkata, India, by explaining the methodology and providing a profile of the Quarantined Student-Youth Network (QSYN). This section also presents data from ethnographic fieldwork on QSYN in Kolkata and establishes how politics of care are operationalised through solidarity networks. Drawing on these data, the conclusion section by summarising the argument provides an alternative framework to theorise care in a postcolonial context.

Infrastructure, Care, and Solidarity Networks During the Pandemic

Continuing from the introductory section, this section critically engages with scholarly work around infrastructure, care, and solidarity networks. It also shows how a holistic understanding of these three thematic areas helps us with a nuanced understanding of the politics of care operationalised during the Covid-19 pandemic.

Reimagining Infrastructure

Infrastructure creates its own spatial and temporal logic in cities (de Boek, 2012). Doing so makes the materiality of interconnected networks that mediate urban space through a complex socio-technical process (Graham & Marvin, 2002). Hence, when we look at infrastructure, it is also important to see how material infrastructure translates to collective social imagination. Popular imaginations around infrastructure predominantly focus on how certain physical structures and facilities enable the smooth functioning of society in general. This framework for understanding infrastructure is modernist. It has also contributed to a colonial expansion of power where the provision of infrastructure was used as a tool for discipline and dominance over the colonised subjects (Chattopadhyay, 2012). However, in the literature on infrastructure, it is often ignored how the provision and access to infrastructure are also shaped through social, environmental, and political parameters. Hence, the critical aspect of infrastructure lies in how certain socio-spatial relations enacted in urban space influence the "making" of infrastructure and vice versa (Steele & Legacy, 2017). It is also important to highlight the simultaneous visibility and invisibility of infrastructure. de Boek (2012) argues invisibility of certain infrastructures simultaneously creates possibilities for a relational understanding of urbanity and hinders the possibility of certain social interactions.

Taking forward that argument, we establish the idea of infrastructure through its invisibility. By invisibility, we do not mean inadequacy of certain infrastructures; we mean forms of networks which challenge the normative discourse around the physicality of infrastructure making. Invisibility also counters the accumulation of surplus capital through the socio-technical networks of service provision. We acknowledge Chattopadhyay's (2012) framing of infrastructure in this regard. She states "Its deviance resides in its nonrecognition in the eyes of the state. This is not just refusal but the inability of the state to comprehend these structures of exchange and linkages within its own logic" (p. 248).

For Chattopadhyay (2012), "infra-making" is dependent on socio-cultural relations and practices. It is also important here to highlight Simone's (2004) work on "people as infrastructure". In "people as infrastructure", he focuses on social collaborations through multiple, iterative everyday acts by people, which contributes to the production of spatial relations (Simone, 2004). These everyday acts are ad hoc or quasi legal, outside any formal institutional framework, and thus generative. They continuously unsettle existing categories and hence with their simultaneity become part of infra making and unmaking (Ray, 2020). This chapter uses this framework of infrastructure to explore during the pandemic how solidarity networks, through their everyday acts, formulate an alternative understanding of reimagining infrastructure. The continuous making and unmaking of infrastructure were more visible during the pandemic, which is discussed in the next section.

Covid Crisis and Politics of Care

The recent pandemic has put forward the idea of reimagining infrastructure, enabling us to think beyond the normative notion of materialistic infrastructure for two reasons. First, due to the uncertainty, continuous spatiotemporal ruptures were created. Second, reduced mobility and social distancing altered the socio-spatial materiality of infrastructures (Lambert et al., 2021). The vulnerability and paradox of infrastructures were more visible through their simultaneous presence and absence in cities. The efforts of the formal sector and frontline health care workers during the pandemic have been well documented (running public transportation system, developing vaccines and caring efforts) (Sanger et al., 2020). However, the work of actors and organisations outside the frameworks of the state and the private sector have been under-documented. It is also important to highlight that the crisis heightened the sense of solidarity among people (Acuto et al., 2020). Though state control and capital accumulation became pivotal in shaping everyday life, the crisis during the pandemic re-established the act of reciprocity and community participation to provide care to vulnerable communities (al Siyabi et al., 2021; Springer, 2020).

It is also important here to highlight how we define care. Care can be conceptualised as a political project which is practised through community solidarity (Power & Williams, 2020; Raghuram, 2012). It is also argued that care is a mobile practice which continuously unsettles the boundary between the caregiver and receivers (Middleton & Samanani, 2021; Raghuram, 2012). Care also highlights a sense of responsibility and becomes an essential part of ethical living (Raghuram et al., 2009). If we map care spatially, it also morphs into a relational interdependence of spaces (Raghuram et al., 2009). Following Massey's (2004) theorisation, McEwan and Goodman (2010) argue care is also represented through mutual connectivity among apparently distant subjects. They also mention often we focus much on the economic value of care. By doing so, the emotional labour often gets unaccounted, though caring work involves a massive amount of emotional labour (McEwan & Goodman, 2010).

There is a resurgence in acknowledging care work during the crisis. However, in many cases, this recognition is merely a symbolic gesture (Schwiter & Steiner, 2020). In many cases across the globe during the pandemic crisis, the state created a popular discourse where they presented themselves as champions of providing and acknowledging care work. This kind of popular discourse can be seen in the campaign "Clap for Carers" in the UK, flowers were showered on doctors by the Indian Armed Force, etc. This shows a pervasive attempt by the state to capture care work and has become an apparatus for demonstrating a nationalistic sentiment. Raghuram et al. (2009) encourage us to look beyond formal sites of care. They ask us to focus on "distant others" whose praxis and modes of living are influenced by neocolonialism (Raghuram et al., 2009). Hence, we need to look at the "undisciplined politics of inhabitation" (Lancione & Simone, 2020: 2). "Undisciplined politics of inhabitation" helps us acknowledge and recognise care practices outside the formal institutional set up. It gets operationalised predominantly by self-organised solidarity networks.

Solidarity Networks

Kropotkin popularised mutual aid as an anti-hegemonic solidarity network in the early 20th century. The Covid crisis has re-established the importance of mutual aid, which can be defined as collective coordination to meet each other's needs (Spade, 2020). This concept may not seem revolutionary as it is true that people have worked together to survive for all human history. Community based approaches for providing infrastructures existed before the pandemic (Yap et al., 2021). Furthermore, charity, aid, relief, and social services have dominated the mainstream understanding of how to support people in crisis. However, Spade (2020) emphasises that solidarity in mutual aid fills the gaps and eradicates the issues created by traditional responses, transcending charity. The notion of charity echoes a utilitarian and rationalist approach to crisis management, typically relying on the elite few to make decisions about providing support to those marginalised and vulnerable. Charity follows strict processes of decision-making and categorisation to determine who gets help, what the limits are to that help, and what the conditions are for receiving it. In contrast, mutual aid is more than charity's unidirectional relationship between the "carer" or the "expert" and "cared for", and instead mobilises knowledge possessed by many people, particularly those who experience the painful realities of crises, and ultimately cultivates a shared analysis of the root causes of crises, poverty, and inequalities.

The state and capitalism have worked in harmony to destroy mutual aid throughout history, particularly through the imposition of private property (Springer, 2020). Rather than strengthening community capabilities, the state has sought to replace bonds based on humanity and emotional involvement with unequal distribution of benefits and subsequent tension and marginalisation across societies. Drawing on results from virtual ethnographies exploring gender relations during the Covid-19 lockdown in Italy, it was found that, in response to intensifying unequal domestic arrangements of parenting duties, many working mothers found creative ways to care for others and themselves (Manzo & Minello, 2020). This included the development of digital connections, such as Zoom parties for children's birthdays, lunches with lonely family members, catch-ups with old and new friends, and the formation of emotional support groups on WhatsApp. These women-centred mutual aid models show that caring is a distinctive, network-based activity that relies on many people to organise care where inequalities are rife. Solidarity extends beyond caring for those involved in kinship relationships (the family and household) and includes relationships between strangers, volunteers, migrants, refugees, professionals, markets, economies, states, and non-human life across the world. Chatzidakis et al. (2020) describe this type of care as "promiscuous" in that anyone can potentially care for, about and with anyone. The indiscriminate nature of such solidarity networks is particularly important for strengthening the provision of services and infrastructure to ensure equitable distribution, including to those marginalised and vulnerable individuals and groups in societies.

This chapter focuses on one kind of solidarity network that was organised during the pandemic and operated outside the formal institutional networks. In this chapter, we aimed to analyse how politics of care was operationalised during the pandemic by one such network. The following section first explains the methodology that was followed for the research. It then contextualises the study in Kolkata by integrating data from the QSYN network.

Contextualising Care During the Pandemic in Kolkata

In our research, we conducted six-months of ethnographic fieldwork in Kolkata and interviewed fifteen volunteers who were actively involved with the Quarantined Student-Youth Network (QSYN). We have interviewed volunteers who provided support in Kolkata and surroundings areas, founder members of the network and volunteers who were managing funds and social media activity of the network. We adopted a critical discourse analysis of transcribed interviews. Visual materials were used to triangulate some of the claims. The data generated from this ethnographic study are used to build a coherent argument outlined in this chapter.

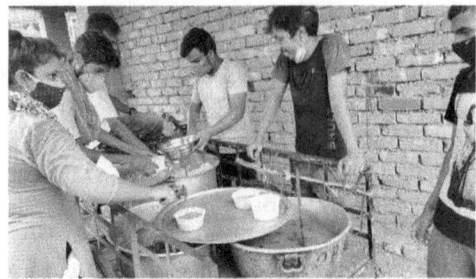 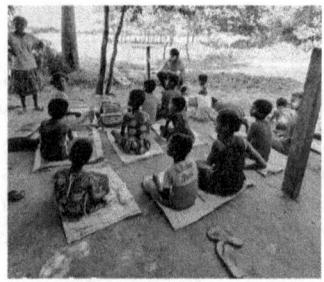

Figure 8.1 QSYN activities.

Source: QSYN.

QSYN is a student-youth led initiative running across Bengal, Delhi, and beyond. Although QSYN started with the onset of lockdown in India as Covid-19 started spreading, an informal network of students existed and re-sponded to social and climate crises like the Nepal earthquake, the Kerala flood, and even after the Delhi riots. A severe lack of support from the state was evident during the crisis, which compelled some of these earlier student networks to form a network for providing support and care to marginalised groups. Currently QSYN has almost 800 volunteers who are engaged in running community-led educational centres for impoverished children, which they call *"Prithibir Pathshala"* (translated to global school). They have almost forty centres across the state of West Bengal (Figure 8.1). During the Covid-19 crisis, they have also run community kitchens. QSYN mainly generated funds from crowdsourcing (both door to door collection and online crowdsourcing) and by organising cultural events.

Amongst many solidarity groups which flourished during the Covid-19 crisis, QSYN is a unique example of operating as a collective and providing care to vulnerable communities.

The analytical part of this chapter is divided into three themes, namely or-ganisational structure, resource mobilisation, and politics of care. The chapter argues why solidarity networks in a postcolonial context can be considered essential infrastructure for providing care to vulnerable communities.

Organisational Structure of QSYN

QSYN operates as a collective of student volunteers. They self-identify neither as a charity nor civil society. In response to our question, a volunteer with QSYN, N[1], told us

> "At QSYN we do not have any formal organisational structure. It is just an informal collective of people who knew each other and have a similar political ideology".

Other members of the group echoed N's statement. They also highlighted that they were already providing support in response to crises even before the pandemic as a collective of students, for example, the Nepal Earthquake Response (2015), Delhi Communal Riot Relief (2020), and Amphan Cyclone Relief (2020). However, on those occasions, they did not identify themselves as a collective nor a network. Instead, they felt they needed to act as responsible members of society and they realised it is a political act for them to respond to those forms of crisis. As the scale and intensity of the pandemic presented a much larger form of crisis, QSYN realised the importance of forming a network. They realised having a formal name and social media presence could help them to mobilise resources that were required during the first and second waves of the pandemic and in the subsequent lockdowns. However, they also saw this as a political act which was not embedded in altruistic relations. For them, "another" just world is only possible through sharing and caring. In turn, they voiced their critique against the state and civil society's responses to the crisis. B, a volunteer in an interview, said

> "The government failed miserably to support poor people during the lockdown. We faced so many troubles in opening our community kitchens. These were by the local political leaders. They wanted to know our affiliations. All the groups we were working with were also victims of harassment by the state".

B also highlighted those obstacles to provide care to the community were not much of an issue. As they were already working with those communities even before the pandemic, their acceptance among the community was higher. Their pre-existing foothold in the community was essential not only for building trust, but also for prioritising their efforts beyond support provided by the state and civil society.

In an interview about A's previous volunteering work during the Amphan Cyclone Relief, A stated

> "NGOs were mainly busy photographing or promoting their work, hence they did not enter the village and observe the situation. When we went there, we did not have any difficulties supporting people as they needed some material help, not the photo opportunities".

A's statement helps us understand how civil society operates as an extension of state power. In doing so, civil society becomes a site for the accumulation of corporate capital (Chatterjee, 2004). While providing packaged food items and hand sanitisers, QSYN faced hindrances both from the state and civil society. In those cases, they decentralised the distribution mechanism by involving local communities. It was easy for them to self-mobilise local communities with their previous presence in that area. QSYN also worked horizontally where there were no pre-defined roles and responsibilities. On some occasions, a volunteer would manage communications channels including social media whilst another volunteer would be busy cooking in the community kitchen. QSYN operationalised need-based work which Spivak calls "strategic essentialism" (Spivak, 2012).

The decision-making process within QSYN is a collective process. They have called general body meetings with all volunteers for decision-making and have also involved the community in the process. When we asked how they decided which would be the site to set up a community kitchen, B replied

"Where should we cook? The place was not a problem. The place was not a problem. The kitchen in the College Street area is the backyard of one of the persons from the community. He went with us grocery shopping, and when we were discussing where should we cook, he said to use his backyard. The pandemic taught us it is all about cooperation. It is not that we are providing food, and they are the beneficiaries."

The above statement from B also highlights how QSYN operated beyond the binary models of care-receiver versus caregiver. The fluidity of this boundary and collective action helped them to reach a broader community and enabled them to navigate within a complex political network locally. QSYN also built resource mobilisation strategy on the principles of collective actions which is discussed in the next section.

Resource Mobilisation

QSYN developed various methods for resource mobilisation at various spatial scales. They have tactically used digital resources and non-digital modes for mobilisation and outreach. A heterogeneous set of actors was engaged in resource mobilisation through a networked mobilisation of power (Allen, 2009). This networked mobilisation is embedded in the principles of emancipation and social change, where each actor has the autonomy for mobilisation (Featherstone, 2008; Papaioannou, 2014). By adopting this strategy of "networked mobilisation" QSYN developed a digital map-based reporting process (Figure 8.2). With the help of this reporting process, the community could self-report where they needed support.

Acknowledging the lack of digital literacy among communities, QSYN also relied on WhatsApp and phone calls for self-reporting. To make the process transparent, they continuously published procurement details and geographical locations where they are providing support to the communities (Figure 8.3). In our interview, N said

"At one point, we were receiving hundreds of phone calls or WhatsApp messages every day. We knew that everyone would not be able to locate their village on the map. However, we updated all those data coming from the phone calls or messages on the map. It helped us also to make the process transparent."

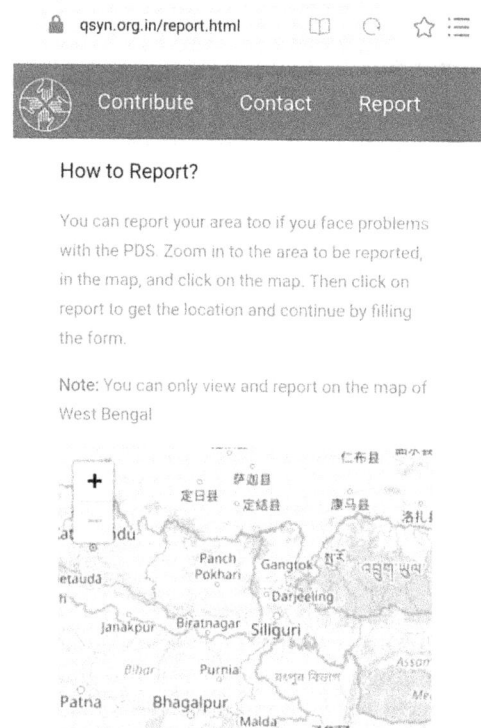

Figure 8.2 QSYN digital map-based reporting process.
Source: QSYN.

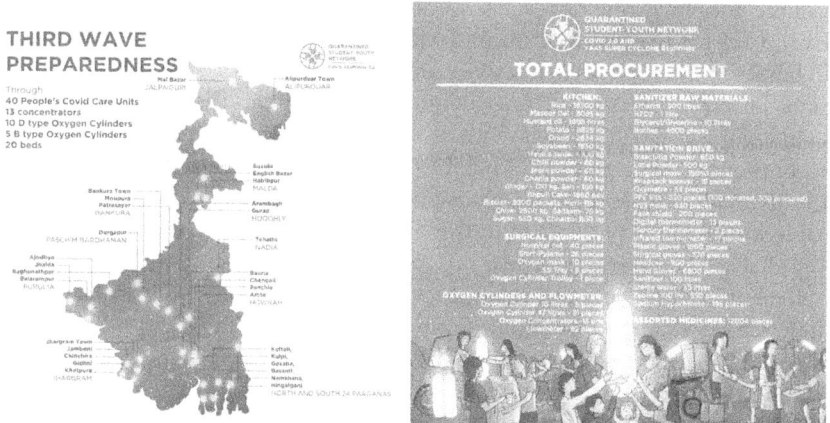

Figure 8.3 Flyer detailing procurement details and support locations.
Source: QSYN.

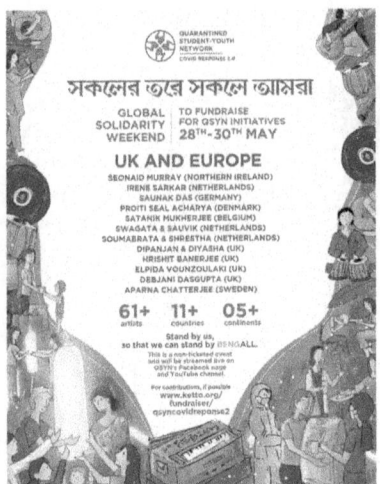
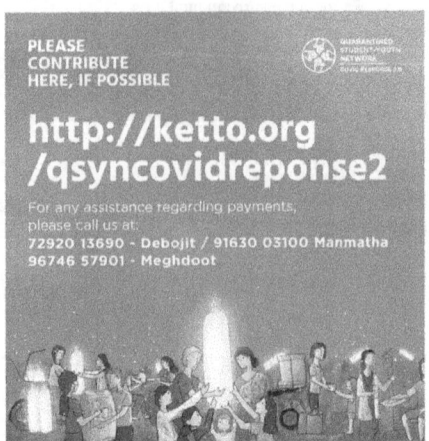

Figure 8.4 Flyer for ticketed QSYN virtual cultural event.

Source: QSYN.

The funding predominantly came from crowdsourcing. QSYN circulated the call for support among diasporic Indian communities across the globe. They also organised a ticketed cultural event virtually and donated all the proceeds to setting up and running their community kitchens (Figure 8.4).

M said QSYN received more than £50,000 (INR 5 million) from Ketto donations (Ketto is an online crowdfunding platform), which they used predominantly to buy groceries and provide personal protective equipment kits to the communities. Community also became an important part of resource mobilisation. On many occasions, the people who pulled hand-driven vans for the distribution of goods were also eating at the community kitchens. They were also involved in prioritising need when there were some surplus materials at one community kitchen; they recommended QSYN volunteers share that with the neighbouring community kitchens. On one occasion, a person allowed QSYN to use his closed warehouse to run *"Prithibir Pathshala"*, and the community repaired that warehouse to enable local kids to participate in the *"Prithibir Pathshala"*. In our interview, M said that the informal nature of QSYN's operation and community involvement in the decision-making process made their model successful. These varied examples of resource mobilisation by QSYN show how collective action is important for solidarity networks for resource mobilisation. Continuing from this, the next section shows how care was provided by QSYN during the pandemic.

Politics of Care

During the pandemic, QSYN provided care in two major forms. In one way, it was running community schools for kids from impoverished backgrounds. In another way, it provided daily meals (for almost 2 years) to the community where the majority of people had lost their jobs and had no money to feed their families. The network started with ten self-motivated students, which grew in numbers within months. As of January 2022, QSYN has almost 600 volunteers across the state of West Bengal. B, in our interview, said that she believed the human urge to help others is the key for QSYN's growth. She also stated that the community was aware that QSYN was neither part of any political party nor working like an NGO. She said

> "We are a network of volunteers where we practiced politics of sharing. The people who were eating in our community kitchens were also involved in cooking, carrying the groceries. They felt it needs to be done by everyone as we are not providing a relief to them".

This alternative space of solidarity which QSYN carved out for themselves, helped them to provide care "differently". B also made it clear in our interview that the lack of political affiliation of QSYN does not mean they are apolitical. Rather, they see care is predominantly a political act, which needs to operate in a non-hierarchical manner that the network managed to establish.

In our interviews, various QSYN volunteers told us that the temporariness and unpredictability of the crisis were so evident that the community's motivation to help others became so effective. As an example, S said when they were in one of the door-to-door money collection walks, a kid came forward and donated £15 (INR1,500), which he had saved for years to buy comic books. S also said it was unimaginable before to see this much solidarity among human beings. The pandemic made people realise how much they need each other for their survival. However, D, another volunteer, said it was not an organic process of realisation. Shared histories and memories of suffering also bound the community together. He stated

> "Most of the people in Kolkata slums are from Sundarban areas. A majority of them migrated recently to Kolkata after the cyclone in the Sundarban area. These are predominantly climate refugees. So, they have history of their own sufferings through their displacement. Hence, they are more sympathetic to people's suffering and try to help others whatever way they can".

S, another volunteer, said for everyone, the motivation was different, and people connected their own struggles with their care work. She cited an example of a girl in her twenties who became a volunteer in *"Prithibir Pathshala"* to avoid her marriage which her family was pushing her to. S[1] stated

"In the village one girl came to us and told us she wants to teach in our Pathshala. Her parents arranged marriage for her as the college is closed and she is not doing anything. She said if she is teaching kids in our Pathshala, she can convince her parents that she is doing some good work. So, she does not want to get married so soon".

These various vignettes from our fieldwork in Kolkata with QSYN show that care work is dependent on mutual human connections. At this juncture, we argue that to understand the politics of care it is important for us to look at the "politics of connectivity". "Politics of connectivity" here means the mutual constitution of distant materiality (Massey, 2004). It operates at a collective level. The data show that even if each member has their own story of displacement, the precariousness of urban living and even the gendered experience of survival (here family pressure for marriage), the pandemic's connected reality compelled them to participate in collective actions. These collective actions can only materialise through a horizontal form of networks that do not operate within institutional frameworks. These networks are ad hoc but simultaneously generative in nature (Ray, 2020). These networks mobilise resources strategically and are based on contextual need and collective actions.

Conclusion

In this chapter, we show how care is operationalised through a solidarity network in Kolkata during the Covid-19 pandemic. The data also highlight how we need to understand care beyond economic terms. We also need to work against the binary materiality of caregiver vs receiver. In the postcolonial context, it is often a fluid subjectivity. Hence, we formulate two propositions in this chapter. First, an alternative theorisation of infrastructure is required. The data show solidarity networks effectively mobilise resources through collective actions for a socially "just world". Hence, we argue for a nuanced understanding of infrastructure through solidarity networks. At this juncture, solidarity networks become an infrastructural apparatus for urban living in the post-colony. By apparatus, here we mean which serves a dominant strategic function at a given time (Agamben, 2009). Second, we argue that care in the postcolonial context is dependent on collective human actions, which operate outside any institutional set up. They are generative as they have possibilities for continuous iterations and unsettle certain normative categories (caregiver vs receiver). Through this framework of care, we also argue for a theoretical category which is "incomplete". Incompleteness as a theoretical category not only helps us to unpack contingent socio-spatial subjectivities of the postcolonial context but also makes theoretical categories generative and relational.

Funding: The research was supported by Global Engagement Fund (UCL) and DPU Internal Grant (UCL). We declare no potential conflict of interest with respect to this research and authorship.

Note

1 Only pseudonyms are used.

References

Acuto, M., Larcom, S., Keil, R., Ghojeh, M., Lindsay, T., Camponeschi, C., & Parnell, S. (2020). Seeing Covid-19 through an urban lens. *Nature Sustainability*, *3*(12), 977–978. 10.1038/s41893-020-00620-3

Agamben, G. (2009). *What is an appatatus? And other essays*. Stanford University Press.

al Siyabi, H., al Mukhaini, S., Kanaan, M., al Hatmi, S., al Anqoudi, Z., al Kalbani, A., al Bahri, Z., Wannous, C., & al Awaidy, S.T. (2021). Community participation approaches for effective national Covid-19 pandemic preparedness and response: An experience from Oman. *Frontiers in Public Health*, *8*(January), 1–8. 10.3389/fpubh.2020.616763

Allen, J. (2009). Three spaces of power: Territory, networks, plus a topological twist in the tale of domination and authority. *Journal of Power*, *2*(2), 197–212. 10.1080/17540290903 064267

Chatterjee, P. (2004). The politics of the governed: Reflections on popular politics in most of the world. In *The politics of the governed: reflections on popular politics in most of the world*. Columbia University Press. 10.3917/mult.045.0174

Chattopadhyay, S. (2012). *Unlearning the city: Infrastructure in a new optical field*. University of Minnesota Press.

Chatzidakis, A., Hakim, J., Litter, J., & Rottenberg, C. (2020). *The care manifesto: The politics of interdependence*. Verso Books.

de Boek, F. (2012). Infrastructure: commentary from Filip De Boeck. *Cultural Anthropology*, 1–10. http://culanth.org/curated_collections/11-infrastructure/discussions/7-infra structure-commentary-from-filip-de-boeck

Featherstone, D. (2008). *Resistance, space and political identities - The making of counter-global networks*. Wiley Blackwell. 10.1111/j.1475-4762.2011.00993_2.x

Graham, S., & Marvin, S. (2002). *Splintering urbanism: Networked infrastructures, technological mobilities, and the urban condition* (Vol. 43, Issue 3). Routledge. 10.1353/tech.2002.0124

Lambert, R., Hoffman, P., & Ray, R. (2021). Infrastructure. In *The DPU (post)COVID Lexicon* (Issue 68). https://www.ucl.ac.uk/bartlett/development/publications/2021/ apr/dpu-news-issue-68 accessed on 1st May 2022.

Lancione, M., & Simone, A. (2020). Bio-austerity and solidarity in the Covid-19 space of emergency - Episode Two. *Society and Space, March*. https://www.societyandspace.org/ articles/bio-austerity-and-solidarity-in-the-covid-19-space-of-emergency-episode-2

Manzo, L.K.C., & Minello, A. (2020). Mothers, childcare duties, and remote working under Covid-19 lockdown in Italy: Cultivating communities of care. *Dialogues in Human Geography*, *10*(2), 120–123. 10.1177/2043820620934268

Massey, D. (2004). Geographies of responsibility. *Geografiska Annaler: Series B, Human Geography*, *86*(1), 5–18.

McEwan, C., & Goodman, M.K. (2010). Place geography and the ethics of care: Introductory remarks on the geographies of ethics, responsibility and care. *Ethics, Place & Environment*, *13*(2), 103–112. 10.1080/13668791003778602

Middleton, J., & Samanani, F. (2021). Accounting for care within human geography. *Transactions of the Institute of British Geographers*, *46*(1), 29–43. 10.1111/tran.12403

Papaioannou, T. (2014). How inclusive can innovation and development be in the twenty-first century? *Innovation and Development*, *4*(2), 187–202. 10.1080/2157930X.2014.921355

Power, E.R., & Williams, M.J. (2020). Cities of care: A platform for urban geographical care research. *Geography Compass, 14*(1), 1–11. 10.1111/gec3.12474

Raghuram, P. (2012). Global care, local configurations - Challenges to conceptualizations of care. *Global Networks, 12*(2), 155–174. 10.1111/j.1471-0374.2012.00345.x

Raghuram, P., Madge, C., & Noxolo, P. (2009). Rethinking responsibility and care for a postcolonial world. *Geoforum, 40*(1), 5–13. 10.1016/j.geoforum.2008.07.007

Ray, R. (2020). *Spatial adhocism as practice for conflict politics: Theorising urban politics in Kolkata.* The Open University.

Sanger, D.E., Kirkpatrick, D.D., Wee, S.-L., & Bennhold, K. (2020, March 19). Search for coronavirus vaccine becomes a global competition. *The New York Times.* https://www. nytimes.com/2020/03/19/us/politics/coronavirus-vaccine-competition.html?search ResultPosition=1

Schwiter, K., & Steiner, J. (2020). Geographies of care work: The commodification of care, digital care futures and alternative caring visions. *Geography Compass, 14*(12), 1–16. 10.1111/gec3.12546

Simone, A.M. (2004). People as infrastructure: Intersecting fragments in Johannesburg. *Public Culture, 16*(3), 407–429. 10.1215/9780822381211-003

Spade, D. (2020). Solidarity not charity: Mutual aid for mobilization and survival. *Social Text, 38*(1), 131–151. 10.1215/01642472-7971139

Spivak, G.C. (2012). *In other worlds: Essays In cultural politics.* Methuen.

Springer, S. (2020). Caring geographies: The Covid-19 interregnum and a return to mutual aid. *Dialogues in Human Geography, 10*(2), 112–115. 10.1177/2043820620931277

Steele, W., & Legacy, C. (2017). Critical urban infrastructure. *Urban Policy and Research, 35*(1), 1–6. 10.1080/08111146.2017.1283751

Yap, C., Cocina, C., & Levy, C. (2021). *The urban dimensions of inequality and equality* (No. 01; GOLD VI Working Paper Series).

9 Abortion Care in Times of Crisis: An Autonomous Feminist Model in Latin America and the Caribbean[1]

Mariana Prandini Assis, Oriana López Uribe, Ruth Zurbriggen, and Verónica Vera

Introduction

All over the world, the unprecedented crisis unleashed by the Covid-19 pandemic installed a range of competing narratives about health in general, and sexual and reproductive health specifically. A common narrative around abortion, in both public health studies and the media, is that the profound ongoing health crisis triggered a dramatic transformation in the way that pregnancy termination services are delivered – from highly medicalised, surgical, in-clinic, to more autonomous, with pills, at-home (Romanis & Parsons, 2020). This narrative, however, makes invisible the work of feminist activists, collectives, and networks of abortion accompaniers (*acompañantes*), who for decades have been developing the political imagination and practice of autonomous abortion (Assis & Larrea, 2020).

Self-managed abortion or *aborto autónomo* (as it is commonly referred to in Latin America and the Caribbean) is defined as an abortion where people themselves access the medicines (mifepristone and misoprostol, or misoprostol alone) and use them to terminate a pregnancy outside the formal health system (Erdman et al., 2018). The history of autonomous abortion is one of social experimentation driven by women's concrete need for abortions in a context of profound legal and social restrictions.

In the mid-1980s, the drug misoprostol was registered in Brazil for the treatment of gastric ulcers, under the trade name Cytotec. Brazilian women quickly discovered that the medication caused contractions and bleeding sufficient to cause an abortion (Coelho et al., 1991; De Zordo, 2016). Information about the medication and its abortifacient properties spread throughout Latin America and the Caribbean, where it was and still is readily available in pharmacies in most countries. As a result, the practice of self-managed abortion with pills became popular knowledge.

Scientific documentation of this informal practice (Barbosa & Arilha, 1993; Coêlho et al., 1994) led to the development of consistent studies on the various obstetric and gynaecological uses of misoprostol, which proved to be an essential medicine for reproductive health (WHO, 2005). Many years after

DOI: 10.4324/9781003301905-11

Latin American and Caribbean women had been using misoprostol to self-induce their abortions, professional associations and international organisations produced guidelines and protocols on the use of the medicine for abortion, treatment of postpartum haemorrhage, and other obstetric indications (FLASOG, 2005; WHO, 2012).

In the mid-2000s, taking advantage of the existing knowledge about abortion with pills and the availability of misoprostol throughout Latin America and the Caribbean, feminist activists began to organise several strategies to support those in need of abortion. In that early period, knowledge about abortion with pills was still limited, so activists made use of all information available while at the same time produced novel knowledge themselves. They made the World Health Organisation guidelines their own, but went beyond merely disseminating it, pushing knowledge about abortion with pills and its limits forward, which is what people living in restrictive contexts need to do.

The models of care implemented by activist strategies in the region are varied and have greatly developed over the last decade (Larrea et al., 2021). For example, in 2008, a feminist group launched the first information hotline in Ecuador, and today there are numerous such hotlines throughout the Americas (Drovetta, 2015; Walsh, 2020) and all over the world (Gill et al., 2021). These hotline activities vary according to activists' resources, scale of work, and legal environment. Another common strategy among autonomous abortion activists is accompaniment (*acompañamiento*). The accompaniment model usually involves interaction and support throughout the abortion process, individually or in groups, face-to-face, by telephone, or online (McReynolds-Pérez, 2017; Zurbriggen et al., 2018a; Zurbriggen et al., 2018b). Like the hotlines, the accompaniment model has also proliferated throughout the region and takes on different shapes, scales, and internal structures depending on the social, political, and legal context where it is implemented.

The amplification of these models of care was not the result of chance, but rather a political commitment made by activists organised in collectives and networks that developed and greatly experimented with these models. The decision to disseminate successful strategies within and across national borders was guided by the conviction that feminist models, while breaking with the violent, hierarchical, stigmatising, and cisheterosexist aspects that often characterise many formal health services, are also malleable and adaptable enough to respond to the challenges and needs of each specific territory.

These resilient and flexible feminist models stood tall when the Covid-19 pandemic swept across Latin America and the Caribbean in early 2020. In the first year of the crisis, surely the harshest period in many of the region's countries, there were increased barriers to access abortion and post-abortion care (Pilecco et al., 2021) and the number of unwanted pregnancies grew at concerning rates. In this scenario, the work of feminist activists providing access to autonomous abortion became even more crucial.

This chapter engages the work developed by *Red Compañera*, as one of such activist initiatives. As of 2017, networks of activists relying on accompaniment practices began organising in a regional network, which would allow them to strengthen their actions through solidarity and mutual support. In 2019, a first regional meeting was held, and the Latin American and Caribbean Feminist Network of abortion accompaniers was founded. In early 2020, just before the outbreak of the pandemic, a second regional meeting took place. The year of 2020 was particularly important as the pandemic reinforced the need for closeness, as well as spaces for exchange and collective support. The continued process of relying on feminist meetings and practices, which developed along with the network, has in many ways allowed it to take advantage of distance and online activities to strengthen its approach to regional embodiment. As the pandemic evolved, the Latin American and Caribbean Feminist Network of abortion accompaniers created its collective and public identity. Named *Red Compañera*, this transnational regional network articulates an assemblage of organisations, networks, and feminist and lesbofeminist collectives that accompany women, girls, and other people to have abortions in a safe and caring way, and free of all forms of violence. The network is currently composed of 23 groups located in 15 countries across the region.

Based on our own experiences within the network and on informal conversations with our fellow *compañeras*, this chapter outlines the alternative model of abortion care emerging from our activist practices. The Covid-19 pandemic, instead of dismantling our strategies or disorienting our vision, provided us even more clarity about our interventions in our territories and the world. We argue that the feminist, compassionate, and political model of care emerging from our practices is based upon three principles: i) comprehensive care, ii) direct action, and iii) horizontal power. As such, this model not only responds to people's real and immediate needs, but also prefigures the future of care that we strive for, as communities and political subjects.

Accompanied Abortions and Care during the Covid-19 Pandemic in Latin America and the Caribbean

Prior to the Covid-19 pandemic, there were several barriers to accessing safe abortion, mainly related to the region's restrictive laws and regulations, lack of provision in the cases abortion is authorised, and socioeconomic and racial inequalities. The pandemic deepened some of these disparities, increasing the barriers that already existed and producing a series of new challenges in the context of isolation, mandatory lockdowns, and mobility restrictions (Campos et al., 2020).

Women were at the front line of care work in formal health systems, their communities and families, a gendered burden that greatly increased because of the disruption caused by the pandemic. Many women and people who needed an abortion were forced to self-isolate near aggressors, without the possibility of seeking help or reporting any possible aggression. Others faced job losses and deep economic instability. Access to contraception suffered from drastic reduction across the region (UNFPA, 2020). Many women and people who needed an abortion had difficulty accessing pregnancy tests, ultrasound scans, and essential supplies to confirm their pregnancies and faced collapsed health systems where sexual and reproductive health services were neither prioritised nor recognised as essential.

For instance, at the most critical moment of the pandemic, care for abortion-related pregnancy complications, as well as access to legal abortion decreased dramatically in Ecuador (Surkuna, 2020). In Colombia, municipal health centres closed their physical locations, and others claimed not being qualified to perform abortions (Rosero & Hoyos, 2020). In Brazil, a new regulation further hindered access to abortion care in the case of sexual violence (Human Rights Watch, 2020). And the National Congress of Honduras amended the Constitution to prohibit abortions under all circumstances (Booth, 2021).

However, the regional landscape shifted in more than one direction. In Argentina, the feminist Green Tide (*Marea Verde*) pushed for prioritising abortion law reform, achieving a victory in December 2020 when the Argentinian parliament decriminalised abortion up to 14 weeks (República Argentina, 2021). In 2021, the Mexican Supreme Court of Justice unanimously decided that the criminalisation of abortion was unconstitutional (Suprema Corte de Justicia de la Nación, 2021). And in 2022 the Constitutional Court of Colombia decriminalised abortion in all cases up to 24 weeks (República de Colombia, 2022).

For the feminist networks of abortion accompaniment, the pandemic meant a great increase in the demand coming from women and other pregnant people seeking to interrupt their pregnancies. Amid the diverse context narrated above, the networks made the firm decision not to close the channels of contact or accompaniment with people in need of care at any time or under any circumstances. Acting upon this decision required a twofold move, which included external strategies towards people seeking accompaniment, and internal ones towards fellow accompaniers and their collective spaces. The networks' accumulated expertise and steady work over the previous years (McReynolds-Pérez, 2017) – a feminist sociopolitical engineering assembled to accompany abortions despite criminalisation and stigmatisation – made it possible to respond to the challenge of accompanying in restrictive contexts despite the pandemic.

Externally, the decision to meet the demand for abortions during the pandemic required planning and restructuring of the forms and modalities of accompaniment, adapting to the new restrictions imposed in each country and facing the challenge of collapsed health systems. A series of practical and urgent measures were put in place, such as (i) extending the opening hours of the contact channels; (ii) changing the opening hours to adapt to women's schedules and their privacy limitations; (iii) implementing and reinforcing dissemination campaigns to reach places where accompaniment networks were not known; (iv) adapting face-to-face accompaniment to the online format, offering different options of access via telephone, digital or text messages and other secure messaging applications, and (v) mapping local health systems to identify allies who could help people to have ultrasound scans, post-abortion check-ups, receive care if needed, or even access abortion in cases allowed.

It was particularly complex to halt face-to-face meetings because feminist accompaniment is based upon empathetic encounters between those who accompany and those who seek an abortion (Zurbriggen et al., 2018a; Zurbriggen et al., 2018b). However, we sought to replicate the atmosphere generated by face-to-face meetings "with intelligence, with feminist engineering, with joy, with imagination" in every way possible in the online format, even though "body to body is irreplaceable" (Ruth Zurbriggen, interview).

Internally, meetings among accompaniers were held in-person whenever possible, and when they were not, meetings were adapted to the online format. Regardless of the format, caring for one another never stopped. Security protocols were updated to the new context and work schedules were revised so that the workload would not burden anyone. Efforts to raise funds were strengthened and financial support was ensured for collectives and groups in need. The response to social isolation was feminist inventiveness and solidarity.

Feminist networking at the regional level has already produced a myriad of positive outcomes. It bolsters the actions of networks and collectives of accompaniers on the local level by allowing us to accompany each other, develop joint strategies and collective response to threats and harms, generate spaces for exchange, joint learning, and strengthening of our collective and individual capacities, improve the way we accompany abortions, and strengthen our political actions and public advocacy in our territories. For those of us who are members of *Red Compañera*, the pandemic has made us rethink life and activism, allowed us to consolidate as a regional network and showed us that collective organisation and feminist responses can strengthen even more in times of crisis. In addition, the current crisis has shown us that abortion accompaniment networks are here to stay because the need for safe, caring, and feminist abortions is constant, exists and resists, even amid a global pandemic.

Our Feminist Abortion Accompaniment Model of Care

Crises, be they economic, political, or health-related, are characterised by threat, urgency, and uncertainty (Lipscy, 2020). As such, they cause deep ruptures in established models and practices while also requiring rapid and innovative responses. In this sense, crises highlight the capacity that we and our policies have to adapt to new and unfamiliar scenarios. At the same time, periods of crisis are beneficial in creating conditions that allow us to reflect upon our own practices and identify more clearly and precisely their unique features.

Reflecting collectively on our accompaniment practices amid the pandemic gave us clarity on what are some of the central principles that drive us and our collective work at *Red Compañera*. These principles, which we discuss in detail in the sections below, represent what we have built as a consensus thus far and grounds a model of care that radically differs from that of formal institutions, public or private. While these institutions treat abortion as a *policy* issue – that is, a singular health matter that demands specific guidelines and technical expertise – we frame abortion as *politics,* breaking free from the dominant public health problem paradigm to treat it as a fundamentally contested, aesthetic and affective issue in everyday life.

Holistic Care

In recent years, self-care has increasingly become a dominant frame for describing self-managed abortion practices (Vázquez-Quesada et al., 2020; WHO, 2019). As such, self-managed abortion has been described as a health experience where people take charge of their own care, autonomously and affirmatively. While the practices developed by feminist autonomous abortion networks and collectives have also been qualified as self-care (Bercu et al., 2021), we understand that the model of care set in motion by our practices is radically different from the dominant care and self-care approaches in the public health field.

Our accompaniment practices fracture the traditional logic in which care is thought of as a unidirectional action or set of actions by the caregiver towards the person receiving care, in a hierarchical matrix of knowledge-power. As such, care practices in the accompaniment model generate other types of relationship characterised by circularity of knowledge-power. Our model of care is best described as a social fabric where people and relationships meet at the same level. And although there are many of us, accompanying and accompanied, our social fabric takes into consideration each and every one of those involved, placing them at its centre. The person who wants or needs an abortion becomes an important part of the social fabric of care, but she is not the only one.

The practices of care developed in relationships of accompaniment take as a starting point the singularity of each personal story and desire, and for this reason are framed within strategies that are at once multiple and diverse, situated, and appropriate to each person accompanied. Acts of care in the accompaniment model are never isolated – we practise them in a way that is entangled with what each specific situation requires and attracts in terms of care. Far from consisting of a set of rigid, standardised, and aseptic protocols, we consider care as a concrete practice, a bond generated between people and developed through the actions of the accompanied person, supported by the accompanier (Burton & Trinidad Peralta, 2021).

Our emphasis is on the interconnectedness and interdependence of us all – a model that therefore departs from the usual focus on the autonomous self whose primary value resides in her individual agency. Ours is a system of care where the most valuable unit is precisely the ensemble of all the parts that make up the system. Circularity means that all these parts are linked through relationships established between accompaniers themselves, accompanied and accompaniers, and accompanied themselves.

As accompaniers who accompany in a network, collective work is a political commitment that makes us co-responsible for the care we offer to others and requires that we also recognise ourselves as subjects in need of care. Indeed, we receive care from the people we accompany as well as we develop our care practices among accompaniers. These caring relationships maintaining our social fabric are not transactional, but reciprocal and horizontal, and thus generate a shared sense of connection, solidarity, and complicity.

The internal caring relationships are sustained through diverse collective care practices, such as holding dialogic spaces for accompaniers to process their experiences, debate and critique the practice of accompaniment; accompanying in a network, which allows the network to support the accompanier in case of doubt or difficulty; and managing resources that allow the recognition of the work done by accompaniers who have key roles such as answering first contact lines, e-mails, among others.

Because of all the characteristics discussed above, the care we provide and receive in the political action of accompaniment transcends concerns with physical health and thematises abortion as both a collective and daily event. This allows not only to avoid the isolation that normally surrounds abortion, but also to take it out of the opacity of private life and to frame it as a political and affective act. As Maria Puig de la Bellacasa teaches, "care is an ethical-political question, not only because it is made 'public' but also because it belongs to the collective and appeals to commitment" (2017, p.160).

Our care engineering was designed and structured long before the pandemic, when we made the political commitment to fight against reproductive injustice in our territories. To this end, we have developed a complex structure of holistic care, designed to enable collective action, and based on feminist praxis. The traits of our care infrastructure – complex, well-assembled, flexible, and adaptable – ensured our capacity to continue accompanying people in their abortions in a moment of crisis as deep as the Covid-19 pandemic.

Direct Action

When we speak of the practice of accompaniment as direct action, we are referring to the political decision to make ourselves available, create time for listening, and encourage the exchange of ideas and experiences in the process of accompanying those who engage with us. Direct action seeks to provide security to those who have abortions and those who accompany them. In other words, it means being there for those who have abortions, to give course to the desire and the need to abort, a form of being that is always collective. Being there to collaborate in reaffirming the decisions taken, subtract fears and shame, so that abortions are removed from the risk of unsafe secrecy. Being there to take care of life and health.

Direct action is made of the availability to offer spaces that provide updated and validated information, support people emotionally and offer relief before the decision is taken. This reflects a circular framework free of prejudices and demands of causalities or motivations. Direct action is also based on laborious engineering that emphasises the planning and organisation of all the steps to be taken with those who are going to have an abortion, seeking to focus on the singularities of each person while recovering what has been done with others who have already had an abortion and shared their experiences with accompaniers. This engineering avoids the labyrinths and bureaucratisation of the formal health system, which is the mirror through which we look at ourselves to be different.

At the same time, direct action is done in and with the corporal territory of those who accompany and those who are accompanied, through theories and practices of the body to body that produce community health. The theories and practices developed out of our direct action are fed by continuous reflections so that the accompaniments put into action the learnings and common goods accumulated in the horizon of humanising all the dimensions involved in an abortion.

Although it confronts formal institutions, our direct action also seeks to have an impact on public policies and state regulations. Indeed, it is committed to changing regulations that criminalise abortion because we are interested in ensuring access – wherever it may be – free of violence, stigma, and denial. We recognise states and governments' debt to autonomy and bodily decisions. Because we are interested in collecting these debts, we demand the total decriminalisation of abortion and contribute to remove the negative burden placed on abortion when it is criminalised in our penal codes but allowed only in certain circumstances and/or up to a certain number of weeks.

Ours is a direct action that prefigures another social and political culture when talking about abortions and demanding legislative changes, because these demands are made from the vital and common experience of accompanying. We project and develop alliances with other organisations so that states recognise people's right to have an abortion, because this recognition produces symbolic and material effects in concrete lives. The direct action we develop does not shy away from seeking solutions to a problem that presents itself in the here and now.

Finally, ours is a direct action that advocates for other sensitivities regarding abortions. Moving certain structures even within feminisms, we aim to rediscuss the senses of right and wrong when deciding to abort and to accompany. This critical discussion engages the terms in which abortions are often thought of such as aspirations centred on faith in the state, the fact that abortion is a public health problem, and the levels of pathologisation with which the issue is often approached. In a non-complacent way, our direct action engages and disputes meanings considering those who abort as people with the power to decide when a life will or will not be, as argues Laura Klein (2013). In short, it is direct action that moves us to accompany abortions to produce other words; words that make it clear that all people who have abortions, regardless of age, gender, sexuality, class, or race, deserve to live that decision as part of creating acts of justice and dignity in their own lives.

Horizontal Power

To transform the way in which we receive and give care, support and respect during abortions is to be constantly critical of the practices we have as a society. As abortion accompaniers, we are facilitators of knowledge and tools but never decision makers. Through our accompaniments, we seek to transfer information, knowledge and denaturalise hierarchical processes and relationships that societies have normalised in the health field, where medical staff often decide what contraceptive method you should use, how your abortion should be, how your pregnancy will be terminated, when the caesarean section will take place, and when you can decide that you do not want to have (more) children. Abortion accompaniers seek to break with medical paternalism that jealously guards its technical knowledge and does not offer options but gives unappealable decisions.

As accompaniers, with an emancipatory intention, we offer our knowledge, time, and experiences for the benefit of those who are having an abortion. This way, people having an abortion know and recognise themselves as the centre of the experience, deciding with whom to share, in what space to be, at what moment to carry out their process and having at hand a network of people who are there to listen to what they want or need to share. As accompaniers we do not ask for confessions or explanations for the decisions made, neither for the decision to abort nor for deciding not to use contraceptives, nor for anything that is or is not related to abortion – throughout the experience all we do is to offer unapologetic feminist support.

We know that being accompaniers places us in a different position of power compared to that of the people who are being accompanied. However, throughout the process we look for ways to erase that difference by generously sharing our knowledge, showing our own vulnerability, and making our doubts and limitations transparent, striving to generate a relationship between equals. Equals because we are all different and authentic, but also because we all face a system that seeks to isolate, separate, and oppress us.

Accompaniers do not seek to replace, duplicate, or mimic the medical figure. On the contrary, from the space of the non-medical we aim to share health, build social tissue, be there for others. In addition, we build a social fabric with medical personnel who seek other ways of doing medicine, ways that are less vertical, built less from morality and more from ethics. With these types of allies, we build a more complete and stronger social fabric.

The networks, collectives and organisations that are part of the *Red Compañera* carry out a task of permanent training to engage more and more accompaniers, so that those who abort can accompany others, so that those who seek to transform the world from feminist accompaniment have tools that in turn reach others. Different from most medical experts, we are not jealous or protective of our tools, strategies, and knowledge. On the contrary, we seek better and more effective ways of disseminating them, always sharing from the principle of placing people who abort not below, not to the side, but at the centre.

Conclusion

In this chapter, we argue that the practices developed by abortion accompaniers such as ourselves in the *Red Compañera* build an alternative model of care based on three principles: i) holistic care, ii) direct action, and iii) horizontal power. This model of care, radically different from models that prevail in formal health systems, reveals our high degree of organisation and commitment to a world different from the one we inhabit today. For us, it is imperative that abortion is framed from the perspective of care communities. By doing so, we build societies that acknowledge each person as fundamental and complete, thus able to decide what is best for their lives if they have beside them a community that provides information, tools, and support so that abortions are no longer taboo and unnecessary risks are no longer taken.

Moreover, this model of care is not simply an abstraction or an aspiration of what we want the world to be. On the contrary, we put into practice the future we desire while living that future today, along and with each accompaniment. In this sense, ours is a prefigurative politics, understood as politics that "model or prefigure a future society at a micro level with the aim to instantiate radical social change in and through practice" (Törnberg, 2021, p. 83). We insist: Autonomous abortion is not another option of a neoliberal system that makes us responsible in a vacuum and isolates us from our communities. On the contrary, autonomous abortion is a reality of organisational, feminist, anti-neoliberal, horizontal, and care work, whose core values we strive to disseminate throughout society.

Note

1 All authors equally drafted, contributed to, and reviewed this chapter and share joint first authorship. Oriana López Uribe, Verónica Vera and Ruth Zurbriggen are founding members of *Red Compañera – Red Feminsta Lationoamericana y Caribeña de Acompañantes de Aborto*, and Mariana Prandini Assis is a collaborator of the network.

References

Assis, M.P. & Larrea, S. (2020). Why self-managed abortion is so much more than a provisional solution for times of pandemic. *Sexual and Reproductive Health Matters, 28*(1), 1779633. 10.1080/26410397.2020.1779633

Barbosa, R.M. & Arilha, M. (1993). The Brazilian experience with Cytotec. *Studies in Family Planning, 24*, 236–240.

Bellacasa, M.P. (2017). *Matters of care: Speculative ethics in more than human worlds.* University of Minnesota Press.

Bercu, C. et al. (2021). In-person later abortion accompaniment: A feminist collective-facilitated self-care practice in Latin America. *Sexual and Reproductive Health Matters, 29*(3), 2009103. 10.1080/26410397.2021.2009103

Booth, A. (2021). Honduras changes constitution to ban abortion. *The Lancet, 397*(10272), 360. 10.1016/S0140-6736(21)00180-X

Burton, J. & Trinidad Peralta, G. (2021). Un aborto feminista es un aborto cuidado. Prácticas de cuidado en el socorrismo patagónico. *Revista Estudios Feministas, 29*(2), e70809. 10.1590/1806-9584-2021v29n270809

Campos, L.S., Oliveira, M.B. & Caldas, J.M.P. (2020). COVID 19: sexual vulnerabilities and gender perspectives in Latin America. *Health Care for Women International, 41*(11–12), 1207–1209. 10.1080/07399332.2020.1833884

Coelho, H., Misago, C., Fonseca, W., Sousa, D., Araujo, J. (1991). Selling abortifacients over the counter in pharmacies in Fortaleza, Brazil. *The Lancet, 338*, 247.

Coêlho, H.L., Teixeira, A.C., Cruz, M.F., Gonzaga, S.L., Arrais, P.S., Luchini, L., et al. (1994). Misoprostol: The experience of women in Fortaleza, Brazil. *Contraception, 49*, 101–110.

De Zordo, S. (2016). The biomedicalisation of illegal abortion: The double life of misoprostol in Brazil. *Hist Ciênc Saúde-Manguinhos, 23*, 19–35. 10.1590/S0104-5970201 6000100003

Drovetta, R.I. (2015). Safe abortion information hotlines: An effective strategy for increasing women's access to safe abortions in Latin America. *Reproductive Health Matters, 23*(45), 47–57. 10.1016/j.rhm.2015.06.004

Erdman, J.N., Jelinska, K. & Yanow, S. (2018). Understandings of self-managed abortion as health inequity, harm reduction and social change. *Reproductive Health Matters, 26*(54), 13–19. 10.1080/09688080.2018.1511769

FLASOG. (2005). *Uso del Misoprostol en obstetricia y ginecología. Santa Cruz de la Sierra.* http://www.codajic.org/sites/www.codajic.org/files/Uso-de-misoprostol-en-obstetricia-y-ginecología-FLASOG-2013.pdf

Gill, R.K., Cleeve, A. & Lavelanet, A.F. (2021). Abortion hotlines around the world: a mixed-methods systematic and descriptive review. *Sexual and Reproductive Health Matters, 29*(1), 1907027. 10.1080/26410397.2021.1907027

Human Rights Watch (2020). *Brazil: Revoke Regulation Curtailing Abortion Access.* Available at: https://www.hrw.org/news/2020/09/21/brazil-revoke-regulation-curtailing-abortion-access

Klein, L. (2013). *Entre el crimen y el derecho: El problema del aborto.* Plural Editores.

Larrea et al. (2021). Medical abortion provision and quality of care: What can be learned from feminist activists? (2021). Medical abortion provision and quality of care: What can be learned from feminist activists? *Health Care for Women International,* 1–20. Advance online publication. 10.1080/07399332.2021.1969573

Lipscy, P. (2020). COVID-19 and the Politics of Crisis. *International Organization, 74*, 1–30. 10.1017/S0020818320000375

McReynolds-Pérez, J. (2017). No doctors required: Lay activist expertise and pharmaceutical abortion in Argentina. *Signs, 42*(2), 349–375. 10.1086/688183

Pilecco, F.B. et al. (2021). Abortion and the COVID-19 pandemic: Insights for Latin America. *Cadernos de Saúde Pública, 37*(6), e00322320. 10.1590/0102-311X00322320

República Argentina (2021). *Ley N° 27.610 – Acceso a la Interrupción Voluntaria del Embarazo (IVE).* https://www.boletinoficial.gob.ar/detalleAviso/primera/239807/20210115

República de Colombia. Corte Constitucional (2022). Sentencia C-055-22. https://www.corteconstitucional.gov.co/comunicados/Comunicado%20de%20prensa%20Sentencia%20C-055-22%20-%20Febrero%2021-22.pdf

Romanis, E.C. & Parsons, J.A. (2020). Legal and policy responses to the delivery of abortion care during COVID-19. *International Journal of Gynecology and Obstetrics*, *151*, 479–486. 10.1002/ijgo.13377

Rosero, C. & Hoyos, G.P. (2020). *Monitoreo de Políticas de Salud Reproductiva en el Marco de las Respuesta al Brote de Covid-19 y Acciones de Incidencia a Nivel Nacional para Fortalecer el Acceso a Servicios Esenciales de Salud Reproductiva a Nivel Nacional (Colombia)*. https://saludreproductivavital.info/wp-content/uploads/2020/12/COLOMBIA.-MONIT OREO-DE-POLITICAS-DE-SALUD-REPRODUCTIVA_02.pdf

Suprema Corte de Justicia de la Nación (2021). Sentencia. Acción de Inconstitucionalidad 148/2017. https://www.scjn.gob.mx/sites/default/files/proyectos_resolucion_scjn/documento/2021-08/AI%20148.2017.pdf

Surkuna (2020). *Monitoreo de políticas de salud reproductiva en el marco de respuestas al brote de COVID-19*. https://saludreproductivavital.info/wp-content/uploads/2020/12/ECUA DOR.-FINAL-la-salud-es-vital-2020-2.pdf

Törnberg, A. (2021). Prefigurative politics and social change: A typology drawing on transition studies. *Distinktion: Journal of Social Theory*, *22*(1), 83–107. 10.1080/160091 0X.2020.1856161

UNFPA (2020). *El Impacto de Covid-19 en el Acceso a los Anticonceptivos en América Latinay El Caribe: Informe Técnico*. https://lac.unfpa.org/sites/default/files/pub-pdf/informe_tecnico._ impacto_del_covid_19_en_el_acceso_a_los_anticonceptivos_en_alc_1.pdf

Vázquez-Quesada, L. et al. (2020). Abortion self-care: A forward-looking solution to inequitable access. *International Perspectives on Sexual and Reproductive Health*, *46*(1), 91–95. 10.1363/46e1420

Walsh, A. (2020). Feminist networks facilitating access to Misoprostol in Mesoamerica. *Feminist Review*, *124*(1), 175–182. 10.1177/0141778919888070

World Health Organization (2005). *Model Lists of Essential Medicines*. http://whqlibdoc.who.int/cgi-bin/repository.pl?url=/hq/2005/a87017_eng.pdf

World Health Organization (2012). *Safe abortion: Technical and policy guidance for health systems* (2nd edition). WHO Press. https://apps.who.int/iris/handle/10665/70914

World Health Organization (2019). *WHO consolidated guideline on self-care interventions for health: Sexual and reproductive health and rights*. https://apps.who.int/iris/bitstream/handle/10665/325480/9789241550550-eng.pdf

Zurbriggen, R., Keefe-Oates, B. & Gerdts, C. (2018a). Accompaniment of second-trimester abortions: The model of the feminist Socorrista network of Argentina. *Contraception*, *97*(2), 108–115. 10.1016/j.contraception.2017.07.170

Zurbriggen, R., Vacarezza, N., Alonso, G., Grosso, B. & Trpin, M. (2018b). *El aborto con medicamentos en el segundo trimestre de embarazo: Una investigación socorrista feminista*. La Parte Maldita.

10 Clash of Cultures: Bureaucracy Meets Localism, Informality, and Trust in Responding to the Covid-19 Crisis in Cape Town

Manya van Ryneveld, Eleanor Whyle, and Leanne Brady

Introduction

Cape Town Together (CTT) emerged in early March 2020 as a neighbourhood-level, bottom-up response to the Covid-19 pandemic in Cape Town, South Africa. The impetus behind it was to build a community-based network that would spread faster than the virus itself, enabling and encouraging people to self-organise within their communities and in solidarity with others around the city. CTT connected neighbourhood-level Community Action Networks (known as CANs) throughout the city to allow for the mobilisation and sharing of local knowledge, resources, and inspiration to tackle real-world challenges of the pandemic and ensuing lockdown.

Despite its progressive constitution, South Africa is one of the most unequal countries in the world, and the country's system of social protection has significant gaps (Francis & Webster, 2019; Lund & Budlender, 2008). In this context, the city of Cape Town is particularly unequal and deeply divided. In the face of a top-down, initially militarised pandemic response from the South African state, networks of mutual aid and support such as CTT played an important role in the pandemic response (Bailie, 2020; Levine & Manderson, 2020; Van Ryneveld et al., 2022). Through a combination of trust-based accountability, horizontality, autonomy, and relationship-building, the CANs present an effective alternative to dominant models of crisis-response in public health emergencies. This unique structure enabled a degree of rapidity and flexibility that enabled the CANs to work alongside formal health system and civil society response efforts and meet the emergent local needs that would otherwise have been neglected. However, in many instances the informal and relationship-driven approach to organising that enabled the CANs to be so responsive to local needs, presented an intractable barrier to working with or getting support from more established organisations, including the state. This chapter reflects on the experience of CTT, drawing out insights regarding how the state's pandemic response can interact with informal and community-led responses to promote and protect the health of the public, and the challenges inherent in doing so.

DOI: 10.4324/9781003301905-12

The chapter is structured into three sections. The first section provides some background to the social and structural make up of Cape Town as a city, highlighting specific issues such as the deep-rooted inequality, progressive but inadequate welfare infrastructure, and a legacy of spatial apartheid. The second section presents three projects that have arisen from the network over the course of the pandemic – a large network of community kitchens, CTT's involvement in the provincial Department of Health's communications strategy, and the "EMS Vaxi Taxi" project, which saw CANs collaborating with Emergency Medical Services (EMS) to launch a mobile, door-to-door vaccine campaign. In the last section, we put forward an analysis of these cases, paying attention to short-term challenges and long-term shifts in perspective, and what this says about countering power imbalances and hierarchical bureaucratic culture to allow for a more people-centred pandemic response.

Context and Background

Cape Town is the oldest and one of the largest cities in South Africa (Sinclair-Smith & Turok, 2012). It is widely regarded as a city of extreme disparities in wealth and socioeconomic status (Turok et al., 2021). Most neighbourhoods remain segregated along race and class lines, often with large distances and physical barriers such as mountains, nature reserves, highways, golf courses, industrial areas, and railway tracks, between them (Sinclair-Smith & Turok, 2012; Turok et al., 2021). Thus, the city contains a huge concentration of wealth in its more affluent suburbs, which exist alongside more densely populated informal and semi-formal neighbourhoods that house most of the city's population but remain under-resourced and under-serviced. Many families, designated Black, Coloured, or Indian during apartheid, were forcibly removed to these areas from other parts of the city under the Group Areas Act of 1950, and the legacy of this spatial apartheid still runs deep in the city today.

South Africa is governed through three spheres of government – national, nine provincial governments, and a third sphere of local municipal governments. The provision of public services, in particular health and social welfare, involves all three spheres. The country has a relatively strong but ultimately inadequate social welfare system, based on cash transfers to vulnerable groups (particularly the elderly and those caring for children) rather than delivery of social services, and bolstered by an expansive third sector of civil society groups, non-profits, private donors, and volunteer organisations (Button et al., 2018; Lund & Budlender, 2008; Patel, 2009). In a public policy context characterised by creeping neoliberalism, economic efficiency logics, extensive privatisation, and market-driven social welfare and health policy agendas, there are large gaps in the social safety net, especially for millions of unemployed and under-employed people in a country with an unemployment rate of close to 35% (Statistics South Africa, 2021). Widespread corruption, wasteful expenditure and malpractice within the public sector has been met with deepening compliance culture and a reliance on bureaucratic accountability mechanisms, often dampening the potential for flexibility, responsiveness, and creativity within the formal welfare system – especially during times of change or instability such as the Covid-19 pandemic. In addition, the sense of chronic emergency that millions of Capetonians live with – with regards to access to basic services such as housing, water, food, and security – means that crises such as the pandemic are layered onto an already heavily strained system.

A key driver of the widespread participation in CTT was a long history of community-based activism, self-organisation, and responsiveness, rooted in the struggle against apartheid and, later, in HIV/AIDs activism (Paremoer, 2018). In many working-class neighbourhoods this practice has never been relinquished, due to the continued struggle to access basic services. In other neighbourhoods, the memory of collective struggle and self-organising persisted and was rekindled by the emergence of the Covid-19 pandemic. The wide network of community groups, volunteer organisations, and local non-profit organisations that exists around the city meant that many thousands of people were ready to mobilise together as the Covid-19 pandemic began to take shape. Thus, when a small group made up of social justice activists, public health students, community organisers, and artists, put out the call to action on social media, the response was rapid, and the network grew exponentially.

The CANs in Cape Town

CTT is structured as a horizontal collective of autonomous, decentralised, and hyper-local CANs from across the city. Anyone can start a CAN in their own neighbourhood by creating a WhatsApp group and registering the neighbourhood and a communication liaison person on the CTT database. At the height of the pandemic, in 2020, there was also an option to sign up via an online sign-up form which would then match you with an existing CAN in your neighbourhood or prompt you to start the first one if none existed. Every neighbourhood is different, thus no two CANs operated in the same way. Some built on existing social networks, community groups, and voluntary organisations, but many were built from scratch by people, previously strangers, who connected over a mutual desire to respond to the crisis. At the height of the response there were over 170 CANs operating in neighbourhoods across the city. As the CANs expanded, solidarity between CANs (and therefore across the city) deepened – based on relationships of trust between individuals who otherwise might never have connected.

The kinds of services provided by the CANs varies widely, depending on the specific challenges experienced by each neighbourhood. During the height of the pandemic almost every CAN was involved in some form of food provision, through fundraisers for food voucher distribution, food parcels, or community kitchens and gardens. Levels of food insecurity soared across the city because of a harsh lockdown and many industries having to close, leaving people stranded without work for many weeks (Wills et al., 2020). Food aid from the state was generally in short supply and was difficult to access, involving a bureaucratic process for verification. Thus, neighbourhood-based food aid such as that provided by the CANs was a very important stop-gap measure for extreme food insecurity. CANs facilitated accessible communication and information sharing on the pandemic through weekly "co-learning" sessions hosted online on a wide range of topics from accessing the Covid-19 relief grant to keeping a community kitchen safe and following Covid-19 prevention protocols, and many more. CANs set up pulse oximeter lending libraries for at-home oxygen monitoring. They provided self-isolation support for people with Covid-19, with some CANs even setting up fully operational community care centres (Cruywagen, 2020) offering a safe space for people from crowded households to self-isolate in their own neighbourhoods.

The range of activities taken up across the network were shaped by an overarching ethos of collective action and self-organising. As the network grew, CAN-members began to identify and articulate a set of guiding principles that were eventually captured in a "ways of working" document (van Ryneveld et al., 2020). *CTT Ways of Working* emphasised some of the key features of the network, such as flexibility, localised responsiveness, relational and trust-based accountability, and a redefining of aid as rooted in solidarity, not charity. It also helped to recognise and legitimise the inherently political nature of this work, while at the same time distancing itself from the grandstanding of political parties and figureheads working within a framework of electoral politics and point scoring.

Methods

This paper presents a collective reflective analysis based on personal experience of the authorial team within the CTT Network. The three authors are Health Policy and Systems researchers who have been working within CTT since its inception. In addition, one author (LB) is a clinician and embedded researcher within the EMS in Cape Town. In 2020 and 2021, the authors worked to facilitate and enable cross-CAN communication and information sharing, establishing several CTT projects designed to enable collective reflection, sense-making, and learning from the CAN experience. This included the establishment of the Connecting CANs Fellowship, which provided CAN-members involved in cross-CAN activities with a space for reflection and resulted in the publication of a cookbook and story-archive (Cape Town Together CAN, 2020). In addition, the embedded researcher in EMS acted throughout 2020 and 2021 as a boundary-spanner (Sheikh et al., 2011) between the CANs and the formal health system and has continued to facilitate connections between CANs and the Provincial Health Department.

In this chapter, we present three case studies of collective responses to the pandemic that are led by, or involve, the CANs. These projects can be understood as sites of interaction between the CANs and the formal health system providing insights into the complexity and challenges of this interaction. Data collection consisted of shared reflection sessions, interviews, and participant observation, and was supplemented by communication records such as Zoom recordings and WhatsApp conversation archives. The discussion presented here is based on the collective reflection of the authors. In this reflection, we sought purposefully to focus on the interaction between the CANs and the formal health system, focusing particularly on the elements of this relationship that have sustained beyond the initial Covid-19 crisis and lock-down. In doing so, we hope to reveal the long-term value of community-led crisis response to building health systems that are responsive to the needs of the populations they serve and to strengthening the relationship between the state and the people it serves.

Cases

CAN Community Kitchens and a Kitchen Voucher Program

The CAN community kitchens are an example of radical social solidarity that emerged in the early days of the pandemic when the hard lockdown was announced. Lockdown restrictions left many daily wage earners without work, resulting in extreme food insecurity and families struggling to put food on the table (Arndt et al., 2020; Wills et al., 2020). While there was some food aid provided by the state, this was slow to get off the ground, difficult to access and inadequate to address the scale of food insecurity being experienced as a result of lockdown (Anciano et al., 2020; Davis, 2020; Ekeland, 2022). In Cape Town, the network of CAN community kitchens spread at an exponential rate, responding to the unprecedented levels of hunger being seen in communities across the city – many CAN-members described hunger as "the second pandemic", and saw little hope of relief from the formal pandemic response (Brady & Valley, 2020). While the primary focus of the CAN community kitchens was to provide hot meals for their neighbours, they were also serving more than food. These kitchens, many of them run by women, quickly became social hubs providing a wide range of support for the many challenges of life under lock-down. Kitchens became the spaces where people could access the latest information about Covid, receive support regarding issues of gender-based violence, or pick up photocopied textbooks for home schooling.

Given the informal nature of the kitchens and the fact that many of them had no institutional backing, other than from within their communities, there was a significant threat that they would be closed by the police for disobeying lockdown regulations. With the recognition that these kitchens were an essential lifeline within the pandemic response, kitchen organisers, health system activists, and public servants from the Department of Health co-developed guidance on "how to keep your community kitchen Covid-free". An unofficial decision was made to place the EMS logo on pamphlets as the stamp of approval. This gave the kitchens some legitimacy, as they could be shown to police officers who may otherwise have seen it as their duty to shut down the kitchen. These initial pamphlets later became part of the formal public health guidance for Covid, demonstrating an unusual but participatory approach to public policy.

Kitchens drew on a range of resources to stay open. These ranged from raising donations across CANs, to collaborating with or establishing food gardens that could provide fresh ingredients. While some kitchens were able to provide their service out of piece-meal donations, it was clear that more stable funding would be required if the network of kitchens was to stay open and continue their vital service. Yet many of the kitchens were informal, often emerging spontaneously from someone's private backyard or garage space. Usually, the approach would be for donors to only fund registered NGOs, and this would have presented a major obstacle to the network of kitchens to access funding.

A collaboration between the CANs, and the Western Cape Economic Development Partnership (EDP) and the DG Murray Trust (DGMT), two formal civil society organisations with long-standing links to the Department of Health, was established to experiment with a funding model that relied on networks of trust, rather than paper-based accountability mechanisms, to determine who qualified for funding. This was possible because the nature of the pandemic had momentarily lifted much of the bureaucratic red tape that normally presents a major barrier to accessing resources, funding, and support. The CANs, together with the EDP and DGMT, conducted a mapping exercise to create a record of kitchens across the city. The process by which a kitchen qualified for funding was a phone call to a neighbour who acted as the reference. Since most kitchens were cooking the same food for their neighbours that they were eating themselves, this was an effective approach.

CAN Involvement in Covid-19 Pandemic Communications Strategy

The Covid-19 pandemic communication strategy of the Department of Health is another example of a CAN initiative that highlights the complexities and power dynamics inherent in collaboration between the CANs and the formal health sector. Early in the pandemic, there was a recognition among decision-makers of the need to shape the narrative of the pandemic into one of solidarity and mutual support, and to avoid metaphors of a "war to be fought and won", especially given the rising fear and stigma surrounding Covid-19, and the country's history with HIV-related stigma and fear of testing (Musu, 2020; The Workshop, 2020). In this context, the Department's communication strategy valued public participation and sought to incorporate community perspectives. The communications group was a relatively informal space made up of senior decision makers, including the Communications Director, the previous Head of Department, and the Chief of Operations, which met every Saturday morning for two to three hours to grapple with the complexity of public health messaging on the pandemic.

Input from the CANs was communicated by LB, facilitating reflection on the lived experiences of CAN members in official public health communications.

This cooperation led to a community radio series on the pandemic where, in place of traditional public service announcements, CAN members from across the city shared experiences of how they were dealing with the pandemic, and keeping themselves and their loved ones safe. Later, the CANs were invited into the steering committee of the Social Mobilisation Working Group, a group set up to enable more specific focus on social mobilisation efforts as part of the state's response. This was a significant development given that, ordinarily, only formal organisations are invited to participate – effectively excluding the perspectives of many of the city's grassroots community group and social activists. Despite these examples of progressive change, the initial appetite for inclusive and creative communication strategies sparked by the sense of urgency surrounding the pandemic waned over time. Soon, the Department's response to the pandemic became more procedural and limited by the usual bureaucratic processes, making it difficult to continue to include the perspectives of CANs and other community groups into the communication strategy.

EMS Vaxi-Taxi

The third example is the "EMS Vaxi Taxi", a mobile vaccination project that built on the network of CANs and community kitchens, working with local community leaders to build trust and provide opportunities for vaccination to low-income neighbourhoods by bringing the vaccines to their doors, at convenient times, including weekends and evenings where necessary. At the core of the project was community engagement and a range of social mobi-lisation activities both online (via WhatsApp and Facebook) and walking door-to-door, distributing pamphlets or a "party invite" with official Department of Health logos, with a trusted community member's name and contact number displayed, for people who had questions. These tools allowed for conversations about vaccinations to be held between trusted community leaders, health care workers and community members, both prior to and on the actual day of the vaccination drive.

The EMS Vaxi Taxi project used the networks of trust developed by the CANs and their community kitchens to nurture and develop relationships and trust between EMS and community members. Importantly, this initiative enabled the seeds of bi-directional trust building by increasing the public's trust in the public health system, while also helping to build providers' trust in the public. The EMS context has been characterised by multiple attacks on ambulance crews who have felt increasingly unsafe while delivering emer-gency services to the public (Ntatamala & Adams, 2022). Activities such as the Vaxi Taxi project enabled a "paradigm shift" (W. Philander, personal com-munications, 20th December 2021) where ambulance crews were reminded of the power of collaboration with community groups. In addition to the con-tribution made to the vaccination program, reaching people who may have otherwise been left behind, the Vaxi Taxi project was also an alternative placement for EMS staff with underlying illnesses, which placed them at high risk for severe illness if they contracted Covid-19 or who were on incapacity leave for trauma related to mental health illness due to the high levels of assaults experienced by EMS staff. The Vaxi Taxi was a place of healing for EMS staff who were unable to return to work, where they found a renewed sense of purpose. In addition, the value of this project extended beyond the vaccination program itself, influencing public policy by creating space for trust-building activities between EMS and community groups, and producing an unanticipated positive impact on the psychological well-being of EMS staff.

Discussion

These experiences present some important lessons about what kinds of resources are needed in a public health emergency. However, the experiences of the CANs also offer lessons about how the state pandemic response can interact with informal, community-led responses to promote and protect the health of the public, and the challenges inherent in doing so.

Challenges of Collaboration

One of these challenges can be understood as a cultural clash between the formal, bureaucratised response of the state and the informal, relationship-driven approach of the CANs. To be clear, health systems are social systems with relationships between people at their core, but they are also subject to rules and procedures that can be detrimental to relationship-building (Doherty et al., 2018; Gilson, 2003; Gilson et al., 2011; Marchal et al., 2016). For example, at a meeting with provincial Department of Health officials to discuss how the department could support the CAN community kitchens, the issue of "accountability" proved a sticking point – the forms of social accountability that had proved to be enabling within the network were insufficient with respect to the bureaucratic norms of the Department. For the CANs, relational and trust-based accountability meant that interpersonal trust and a sense of shared goals ensures that resources are used in a way that makes the most sense in that neighbourhood in that moment. For the officials, however, "accountability" meant bureaucratic processes that would ensure resources are used according to pre-determined criteria. Such an approach is not only at odds with the hyper-local, flexible, and informal approach that was core to the operation of many CANs, but would constrain the ability of the CANs to move quickly in response to emerging needs, and in some cases, place an administrative burden that exceeds the capacity of CANs operating with very limited resources.

The CAN kitchen voucher programme is significant because it presents a rare example of a formal organisation recognising the value of informality and modifying its procedures to embrace this approach. While it would usually be necessary to be a registered non-profit organisation to apply for funding to support a community-kitchen, the voucher programme made funding available to unregistered, informal groups as well – in doing so, supporting the CAN community kitchens without imposing accountability procedures that would have slowed progress for some and kept the support entirely out of reach of others.

This type of culture-clash between the bureaucracy of the Department and the informality of the CANs was a recurrent challenge in the height of the pandemic and persists today. Despite a good-faith desire for collaboration on the part of both the CANs and various individuals and Departments of local and provincial government, most opportunities for either transfer of tangible resources or participation in decision-making were stymied by the challenge of different "ways of working".

A second challenge was the politicisation of the CANs and overt efforts to denounce the CANs and their contribution to the pandemic. In the early days of the pandemic, CTT and the CANs were little known and were still developing a collective identity. Over time, however, as more and more CANs emerged and their efforts received increasing attention in mainstream and social media, and as the government's response to the pandemic was increasingly subject to popular scrutiny, the CANs became increasingly politicised.

For example, the then-Mayor of Cape Town publicly denounced the CANs as "a movement that clearly has an alternative agenda" and accused the CANs of misleading caring residents who wanted to help those in need – in a piece accusing a variety of NGOs of encouraging residents to break the law (Plato, 2020). The article cited a clash between the Ward Counsellor and a local CAN in which the CAN – who were renting and had renovated an abandoned and disused community hall to use as a community care centre and food garden – was accused of "occupying" the space illegally (Mayman et al., 2020). There were also reports of instances of government officials being told explicitly not to endorse or work with the CANs.

To a large extent, these tensions were heightened because of the intense focus on the inadequacy of the state's response to the pandemic, and because the CANs served as an exemplar of how much can be achieved quickly and with very few resources. Thus, even as the particular approach of the CTT network made working with the state difficult, this was precisely because it enabled a rapid, flexible and empowering response that was able to respond to emerging needs in a way that many formal organisations, including the state, could not. As the intensity of the pandemic begins to lift and the public's attention is less focused on the shortcomings of the state response, we are beginning to see increasing openness to learning from the experience of the CANs to strengthen the interface between the state and the people it serves. In particular, the value of informal, relationship-driven organising, and, secondly the importance of localism in crisis response is being acknowledged. For example, the Department's recent medium-term Framework for Action strategy speaks of "opportunities … to build a different relationship with communities" and the importance of responding "to the changing priorities and needs of the local population" (Western Cape Government, 2022).

Relationship Building and Localism

CTT began as an informal gathering of neighbours aimed at supporting each other during the pandemic. While some CANs have formalised in an effort to aid fund-raising, many CANs remain entirely informal. Over the course of the pandemic the value of informality and relationship-driven organising – what a lack of structures, hierarchies, and bureaucracy enables – became clear. For example, the CAN community kitchens fulfilled a vital function by serving hot meals to those who found themselves entirely without income during the lockdown. However, by providing a community-based meeting space in which realistic Covid-safe protocols were not only communicated but actively demonstrated, the kitchens also acted as hubs for public health messaging of a new kind. Posters and pamphlets with Covid-safety messaging, which were co-produced by CANs and public health doctors, but which bore official logos, supported this real-world demonstration. Having built relationships through sustained provision of meals that were shared unconditionally and unquestioningly, the kitchens became a hub for sharing trusted information. When these hubs were further used as a launch-pad for the Vaxi-Taxi vaccination days, this trust became an important element in overcoming fears regarding the vaccine. Furthermore, in a context where public health service delivery is often characterised by a failure to deliver quality services in a respectful way, the kitchens presented an important opportunity to regain that trust and strengthen the relationship between the public, the health system, and providers on the ground such as the EMS.

However, the Vaxi-Taxi vaccination days were entirely dependent on the strength of relationships between the EMS programme organisers, the CAN members running the kitchens, and the community members who used the kitchens. These relationships, formed in the early days of the pandemic proved an incredibly valuable resource. At the same time, these relationships allowed the EMS workers to regain a sense of trust in the communities they serve and to begin to overcome the trauma of ambulance attacks. Thus, a key lesson emerging from the experience of the CANs is the public health value of initiatives that enable human relationships and build trust.

A further lesson is the importance of localism in responding to a public health crisis like a pandemic, but also in building responsive health systems more generally. The inclusion of CANs in the Social Mobilisation Working Group represented a rare example of community-members being included in decision-making spaces within the formal health system. Whether this inclusion resulted in a tangible change in public policy or not remains to be seen. However, the inclusion of informal groups in a decision-making space indicates a potential shift toward public policy that recognises the importance of context-specific, appropriate messaging, and the inclusion of voices other than solely those of formally recognised community groups. By helping to get vaccines to people's front doors, the Vaxi-Taxi initiative was another example that demonstrated recognition of the importance of localism from within the formal health system. While the government's vaccination programme was largely facility based, the Vaxi Taxi initiative was one of a couple of initiatives that seeks to meet people where they are, and drew on existing networks of personal relationships and trust to tackle vaccine hesitancy.

Every neighbourhood is different – with different needs and capacities. Knowledge based on lived experiences of the challenges facing a community, and what kinds of solutions are feasible in that particular neighbourhood is vital to an effective pandemic response. Community-level intelligence borne by "Professors of the Street" is a valuable source of data (Whyle et al., 2020). In some neighbourhoods, door-to-door delivery of food parcels might work better than community kitchens. In one neighbourhood a community food garden might flourish, while in another low-quality soil or a lack of space might make such an initiative impossible. In the face of a generalised, top-down and centre-driven pandemic response, the CANs demonstrated the importance of localism, but also highlighted the imperative for government to establish mechanisms to support informal, community-led mutual aid efforts. In a public health crisis, the role of the state should be to find ways to support informal, flexible, localised responses. This requires that public servants be given the freedom and flexibility to learn from and support initiatives like the CANs.

Conclusion

In South Africa, and elsewhere, public policy and pandemic response discourse is peppered with references to "community participation", "innovation", and "responsiveness". In practice, however, organisational hierarchies, power dynamics, and bureaucracy govern the behaviour and choices of the people that make up the formal health system – and in a context rife with corruption and service delivery failures, accountability and efficiency are so often the order of the day. This has led to a compliance culture which, while intended to reduce corruption and ensure appropriate use of the public purse, make supporting community-led initiatives very difficult.

In addition to meeting the emergent needs of thousands of ordinary people in the height of the pandemic, the value of the CANs is that they demonstrate an alternative – mutual aid as an alternative approach to resource distribution, solidarity as an alternative to charity, and embracing informality as an alternative to requiring bureaucratic compliance in the state's crisis response. However, given the hegemonic nature of bureaucracy and hierarchy in public institutions, there is likely to be significant resistance to such change – as was evidenced by the contestation and mistrust with which many actors in the formal health system responded to the CANs.

Nonetheless, the case-studies presented here suggest that, while the intensity of the pandemic, the politicisation of the CANs, and the change-resistant and bureaucratic nature of the formal health system presented significant challenges to the cross-pollination of ideas and resources, these lessons are slowly diffusing, and incremental change is occurring. While a concerted effort to take time to reflect, elucidate, capture, and communicate those lessons from within the network helps, it is, alone, insufficient to bring about a new way of thinking and acting within the state. This experience suggests that the human relationships formed between government officials (at any level) and CAN members enabled the diffusion of ideas from the practice of the CANs into the policy and practice of the Department of Health. The crisis of the Covid-19 pandemic opened a window of opportunity to bypass the constraints of hierarchy and bureaucracy and, instead, to build these relationships, both within the CTT network, and beyond it.

The features of the CANs that enabled them to respond so swiftly and effectively to emerging local needs, also constrained the ability of the formal health system to support their efforts. By embracing informality, focusing efforts at the hyper-local level, and investing in relationships, it is possible not only for the formal health system to support and enable community-led pandemic responses like CTT, but also, in doing so, to strengthen the relationship between the state and the communities it serves. However, to do so will require a concerted effort to loosen the hold of bureaucracy and build flexible, adaptive health systems that can accommodate informality and support bottom-up public health initiatives.

References

Anciano, F., Cooper-Knock, S., Dube, M., Majola, M., & Papane, B.M. (2020, 13 May). Lockdown diaries: The politics of food parcels in Cape Town. *Daily Maverick.* https://www.dailymaverick.co.za/article/2020-05-13-lockdown-diaries-the-politics-of-food-parcels-in-cape-town/

Arndt, C., Davies, R., Gabriel, S., Harris, L., Makrelov, K., Robinson, S., Levy, S., Simbanegavi, W., van Seventer, D., & Anderson, L. (2020). Covid-19 lockdowns, income distribution, and food security: An analysis for South Africa. *Global food security, 26,* 100410. 10.1016/j.gfs.2020.100410

Bailie, C. (2020, 28 May). South Africa's military is not suited for the fight against COVID-19. Here's why. *The Conversation.* https://theconversation.com/south-africas-military-is-not-suited-for-the-fight-against-covid-19-heres-why-138560

Brady, L., & Valley, D. (2020). *Cape Town Together* A. Khanna & R. Desai. https://vimeo.com/481270293

Button, K., Moore, E., & Seekings, J. (2018). South Africa's hybrid care regime: The changing and contested roles of individuals, families and the state after apartheid. *Current Sociology, 66*(4), 602–616. 10.1177/0011392118765243

Cape Town Together CAN. (2020). *Dala Kitchen* (E. Whyle, M. van Ryneveld, & L. Brady, Eds.). Cape Town Together CAN. https://drive.google.com/drive/folders/1Bny7byig5gEfL2_a9Wyj0E5mfazrWksb

Cruywagen, V. (2020, 9 July). Community pulls together to convert creche in Ocean View into a Covid-19 isolation centre. *Daily Maverick.* https://www.dailymaverick.co.za/article/2020-07-09-community-pulls-together-to-convert-creche-in-ocean-view-into-a-covid-19-isolation-centre/

Davis, R. (2020, 17 April). The biggest lockdown threat: Hunger, hunger, everywhere. *Daily Maverick*. https://www.dailymaverick.co.za/article/2020-04-17-the-biggest-lockdown-threat-hunger-hunger-everywhere/

Doherty, J., Gilson, L., & Shung-King, M. (2018). Achievements and challenges in developing health leadership in South Africa: The experience of the Oliver Tambo Fellowship Programme 2008-2014 [Article]. *Health policy and planning, 33*, ii50–ii64. 10.1093/heapol/czx155

Ekeland, M.G. (2022). COVID-19's ambiguous parcel: Agency, dignity, and claims to a rightful share during food parcel distribution in lockdown South Africa. *Economic Anthropology, 9*(1), 137–148. 10.1002/sea2.12224

Francis, D., & Webster, E. (2019). Poverty and inequality in South Africa: critical reflections. *Development Southern Africa, 36*(6), 788–802. 10.1080/0376835X.2019.1666703

Gilson, L. (2003). Trust and the development of health care as a social institution. *Social science & medicine, 56*(7), 1453–1468. 10.1016/S0277-9536(02)00142-9

Gilson, L., Hanson, K., Sheikh, K., Agyepong, I.A., Ssengooba, F., & Bennett, S. (2011). Building the field of health policy and systems research: social science matters. *PLoS Medicine, 8*(8), e1001079. 10.1371/journal.pmed.1001079

Levine, S., & Manderson, L. (2020, 24 August). The militarisation of the COVID-19 response in South Africa. *Medizinethnologie: Körper, Gesundheit und Heilung in einer globalisierten Welt*. https://www.medizinethnologie.net/the-militarisation-of-the-covid-19-response-in-south-africa/

Lund, F., & Budlender, D. (2008). Politcal and social economy of care: South Africa research report 1. *United Nations Research Institute for Social Development, Research Report 1.*

Marchal, B., Van Belle, S., Hoerée, T., De Brouwere, V., & Kegels, G. (2016). *Complexity in Health: Consequences for research & evaluation, management and decision making.* Institute of Tropical Health.

Mayman, N., Whyle, E., Hare, A., & Hayat, G. (2020). Bonteheuwel community group takes flak from DA councillor for their Covid-19 relief efforts. *The Daily Maverick*. https://www.dailymaverick.co.za/article/2020-08-11-bonteheuwel-community-group-takes-flak-from-da-councillor-for-their-covid-19-relief-efforts/

Musu, C. (2020). War metaphors used for Covid-19 are compelling but also dangerous. *The Conversation*. https://theconversation.com/war-metaphors-used-for-covid-19-are-compelling-but-also-dangerous-135406

Ntatamala, I., & Adams, S. (2022). The correlates of post-traumatic stress disorder in ambulance personnel and barriers faced in accessing care for work-related stress. *Int J Environ Res Public Health, 19*(4). 10.3390/ijerph19042046

Paremoer, L. (2018). Situating expertise: Lessons from the HIV/AIDS epidemic. *Global Challenges, 1700076*, 1–11. 10.1002/gch2.201700076

Patel, L. (2009). Thematic Paper: The Gendered Character of Social Care in the Non-profit Sector in South Africa.

Plato, D. (2020, 19 August). NGOs on wrong side of the law, says Cape Town mayor Dan Plato. *IOL*. https://www.iol.co.za/weekend-argus/news/ngos-on-wrong-side-of-the-law-says-cape-town-mayor-dan-plato-84d76218-2fd4-46ca-a613-4685835cda44

Sheikh, K., Gilson, L., Agyepong, I., Hanson, K., Ssengoba, F., & Bennett, S. (2011). Building the Field of Health Sysemts and Policy Research: Framing the Questions. *PLoS Medicine, 8*(8), 1–6. 10.1371/journal.pmed.1001073

Sinclair-Smith, K., & Turok, I. (2012). The changing spatial economy of cities: An exploratory analysis of Cape Town. *Development Southern Africa, 29*(3), 391–417. 10.1080/0376835X.2012.706037

Statistics South Africa. (2021). *Quarterly Labour Force Survey (QLFS) – Q3:2021.* Online: Republic of South Africa Retrieved from http://www.statssa.gov.za/?p=14957#:~:text= The%20official%20unemployment%20rate%20was,2021%20to%2014%2C3%20million

The Workshop. (2020). *How to talk about Covid-19: Narratives to support good decision-making and collective action.* www.theworkshop.org.nz

Turok, I., Visagie, J., & Scheba, A. (2021). Social inequality and spatial segregation in Cape Town. In *Urban Socio-Economic Segregation and Income Inequality* (pp. 71–90). Cham: Springer.

Van Ryneveld, M., Whyle, E., & Brady, L. (2022). What is COVID-19 teaching us about community health systems? A reflection from a rapid Community-Led mutual aid response in Cape town, South Africa. *International Journal of Health Policy and Management,* *11,* 5–8. 10.34172/IJHPM.2020.167

van Ryneveld, M., Whyle, E., Brady, L., Radebe, K., Notywala, A., van Rensburg, R., Mayman de Gras, N., & De Vries, S. (2020). Cape Town together: Organizing in a city of islands. *ROAR Magazine,* 05-05-2020. https://roarmag.org/essays/cape-town-together-organizing-in-a-city-of-islands/

Western Cape Government. (2022) *Health is everybody's business: A framework for action over the 2022 MTEF.* Western Cape Government.

Whyle, E., Van Ryneveld, M., Brady, L., & Radebe, K. (2020). Sparks, flames and blazes: Epidemiological and social firefighting for Covid-19. *Daily Maverick.* https://www.dailymaverick.co.za/article/2020-04-24-sparks-flames-and-blazes-epidemiological-and-social-firefighting-for-covid-19/

Wills, G., Patel, L., van der Berg, S., & Mpeta, B. (2020). *Household resource flows and food poverty during South Africa's lockdown: Short-term policy implications for three channels of social protection.* (National Income Dynamics Study (NIDS) - Coronavrius Rapid Mobile Survey (CRAM), Issue.

11 Psychological, Social, and Political Implications of UK Covid-19 Mutual Aid Groups

Emma O'Dwyer and Luiz Gustavo Silva Souza

Introduction

Grassroots, community-led responses to the Covid-19 pandemic were an essential means by which people were able to survive the pandemic across the world (Carstensen et al., 2021; Sitrin & Colectiva Sembrar, 2020). In the United Kingdom (UK), thousands of "mutual aid" groups mobilised in March 2020 to help their neighbours with the difficulties of the self-isolation imposed by the UK government's "lockdown". Some of these groups had existed prior to the pandemic, developing out of community organisations, parish councils, and other local structures, while others were entirely new initiatives. These Covid-19 mutual aid groups (CMAGs) were essential for the UK population's ability to endure the hardships and difficulties which the pandemic brought (Tiratelli & Kaye, 2020, O'Dwyer, Souza, & Beascoechea-Seguí, 2022). As described elsewhere in this volume (Chapter 7), CMAGs were engaged in many activities in their communities, including but not limited to delivering food and medication, providing social and emotional support through hotlines and "buddy" systems, and providing financial assistance in some cases.

Before proceeding, it is first worth providing a definition of mutual aid. The term originated in the work of anarchist political theorist Peter Kropotkin (1902), who argued that co-operation and mutual aid were as vital (if not more so) for survival, than competition. Mutual aid is a system of horizontal organising to meet each other's needs which is rooted in "an awareness that the systems in place are not going to meet them" (Spade, 2020, p. 7). "Solidarity, not charity" was the slogan of many UK CMAGs (Chevée, 2021) as it counters the unequal power relations embedded in models of charity. From an anarchist perspective, mutual aid does not mean filling the gaps left by the state – it is about creating a new type of society *which actively resists* the authoritarian state. While it should be self-evident that not all members of UK CMAGs subscribed to these values or beliefs, the widespread adoption of this terminology during the pandemic is certainly curious, and raises questions as to the variability in terms of how mutual aid was actually performed (e.g., Mould et al., 2022).

This chapter describes research we have been conducting on the phenomenon of Covid-19 mutual aid groups in the UK since the beginning of the

DOI: 10.4324/9781003301905-13

pandemic, in March 2020. At the outset of this project, we were interested in the *implications* of participation in these groups – psychological, social, and political – and sought to examine them using both qualitative and quantitative methods, using data collected between March 2020 and October 2021. In this chapter, we will shed light on each of these inter-related dimensions by exploring several questions of relevance to Covid-19 mutual aid groups in the UK.

Who Joined Covid-19 Mutual Aid Groups?

We now know a good deal about who participated in Covid-19 mutual aid groups. In April–May 2020, we surveyed over 800 members of mutual aid groups, with participants solicited through social media and the central organising website for mutual aid in the UK – Covid-19 Mutual Aid. Our analysis showed that most participants were white (90%), and their average age was 48 years (range 16 to 78, $SD = 12.91$). In line with other research which has found a greater propensity for women to help others during the pandemic (e.g., Mak & Fancourt, 2021), 84% of participants were female. We also asked questions about socio-economic background and found that 76% were in managerial, administrative, and professional occupations, using the National Statistics Socio-economic Classification (Rose & Pevalin, 2003). Participants were well-educated, with over 60% stating that they had achieved an undergraduate or postgraduate degree. These findings, taken together, portray the membership of CMAGs as relatively privileged economically, and supports other research which has found the over-representation of the groups in areas which had higher scores on wellbeing, social capital, and wealth (Felici, 2020; Tiratelli & Kaye, 2020).

Given the anarchist foundations of the concept "mutual aid", we also asked questions to gauge the political orientation of members. Relative to the general UK population, our participants reported much higher rates of political party membership (19% versus 2%) and reported left-wing political views (4.9 on a 7-point ideological self-placement measure). This suggests that participants in CMAGs were unlikely to be members of the governing Conservative party. Interviews with participants in CMAGs subsequently bore this out – none identified as members of the Conservative party, but many were members of or supporters of the Labour Party, or the Liberal Democrats. Covid-19 mutual aid seems to have been more appealing to those with more left-wing views, but it was *not* a movement of anarchists, as has already been noted and critiqued (Preston & Firth, 2020). Similarly, an early survey of members of UK CMAGs found that members of UK Covid-19 mutual aid groups were interested in politics and willing to engage in political action but viewed their mutual aid activities as apolitical (Wein, 2020).

There are a number of implications of this demographic analysis of the membership of UK CMAGs. First, as we have discussed previously (O'Dwyer, 2020), the over-representation of relatively privileged people in these groups may have lowered the potential for intergroup contact and potentially, solidarity, and may have served to advantage *already advantaged* communities. Second, Zuri (2020) argued that mutual aid was rooted in the communities and experiences of racialised minorities, and that it had been co-opted by white middle-class communities. This issue of the co-optation of mutual aid is a frequent concern (Spade, 2020), having also been discussed in relation to the way in which radical political views were side-lined in UK CMAGs (Preston & Firth, 2020), and the appropriation of mutual aid activities by Conservative MP Danny Kruger (Mould et al., 2022; O'Dwyer, Souza et al., 2022). Mutual aid – what it means and who gets to do it – is fundamentally contested. Third, we have drawn attention previously to the over-representation of women in UK CMAGs and asserted that the UK Covid-19 community response requires an analysis in terms of gender – why were women more likely to help, and what might the consequences of this be in terms of their future political and community participation? (O'Dwyer, Beascoechea-Seguí, & Souza, 2022). Each of these issues are useful areas of focus for future research into community responses to Covid-19, in the UK, and globally.

How did Group Members Understand Mutual Aid?

As mentioned above, the concept of mutual aid originates in anarchist political theory, specifically the work of Peter Kropotkin. While some CMAGs subscribed to an anarchist interpretation of mutual aid, by maintaining independence from state actors (e.g., the police, local council), other groups took a more "service-provision" "apolitical" approach which did not preclude collaboration with these actors if necessary. This led us to question the ways in which mutual aid was understood and enacted by members of UK CMAGs (O'Dwyer, Souza, et al., 2022). Using a social representations framework (e.g., Chapter 1, this volume) and informed by work which has applied this lens to the study of citizenship (e.g., Andreouli & Brice, 2021; Kadianaki & Andreouli, 2015), we sought to explore how members of mutual aid groups conceived of their groups' characteristic values, processes, and relationships with other groups, local structures, and organisations. To examine these questions, we conducted semi-structured interviews with 29 members of UK CMAGs between the 12th May and 3rd June 2020. The data collection period co-occurred with the first period of national "lockdown", which was announced by the UK Prime Minister Boris Johnson on the 23rd of March. Data were transcribed and analysed using reflexive thematic analysis (Braun & Clarke, 2019). We developed three themes from the data, which we describe and analyse below. All participants have been given pseudonyms.

Organised Units

Participants described their groups as nimble and efficient, with their activities facilitated by a suite of web-based tools (particularly WhatsApp,

Zoom, and Google Sheets/Docs). Their groups prioritised getting "people help in the fastest and most efficient way possible" (Sam, 21, Greater London). Across the interviews, the efficiency of CMAGs was frequently worked up by setting up a contrast with the local council, which also had a responsibility for delivering emergency support in communities: "if we'd left it to the local council, they'd still be working out what colour to print the leaflet at the moment" (David, 59, Wales), serving to underscore the efficacy of their groups.

CMAGs were also incredibly complex organisations. Consonant with the anarchist conceptualisation of mutual aid, they were described as non-hierarchical structures. While there were "admins" (Hannah, 26, North West England) or "facilitators" (Katie, 27, Greater London), this was organic and driven by necessity (i.e., the scale of activities or the size of the area covered) and the skills of group members, rather than a desire for power or control by a certain subset of individuals. Furthermore, CMAGs were described as "fluid" (Malcolm, 43, Greater London) and "loose" (Michael, 70, Greater London) and the possibility of moving into different roles within the structure was often emphasised by participants.

An interesting tension was also identified in participants' talk about the structure of their mutual aid groups, as evident in Sam's statement below:

> We have officer teams that are split up between, let me remember, general officers. So, as I said, that's people who coordinate between the different groups. Task officers who collate and then send out tasks to be done by volunteers. Ground officers whose job is to organise our structure and to get new volunteers into the system and to do introduction meetings and all that. Outreach officers, that would effectively be the marketing wing of the group and their job is to coordinate with the council and other groups, and also to expand our reach into the community. I'm forgetting one. There's GDPR, data and finance, and the legal team. But that's just basically compliance.
>
> (21, Greater London)

Participants' talk about their groups in many instances connoted the corporate structure, referencing terms such as GDPR and "outreach". There are two interpretations possible here. The first is that the use of such terminology signified an attempt to anchor mutual aid within a charity model, a framework for delivering aid which works to uphold capitalism and the state (Mould et al., 2022). The other interpretation is that participants used these terms strategically and pragmatically (Changfoot, 2007); their invocation of the corporate sphere denoted resistance to it, signifying an attempt to gain legitimacy for a group which prioritises solidaristic rather than individualistic ways of structuring society. It is possible then that this sort of corporate vocabulary provided participants with the register to claim the efficacy and efficiency of their groups while they simultaneously resisted the type of citizenship it signified.

Mutual Aid Within/Against

Participants frequently critiqued the local government response to the pandemic, and particularly the conditional nature of support provided by local councils. This was contrasted with the trust-first, no questions asked support provided by their groups:

> So, the council's attitude is that people need to be referred to food banks by one agency or another or the council. So that you have to prove you're in need of food and so on. Whereas our attitude and the community kitchen's attitude is if you say you need food then you get food. And it's no questions asked either about sort of whether you really need it or about things like migration status which can be an issue as well.
>
> (Michael, 70, Greater London)

Mutual aid groups "wouldn't see anybody hungry" (Andrea, 51, East Midlands); they provided support irrespective of legal status or "deservingness". This contrast between the work of CMAGs and local government functions as a critique of the highly conditional social welfare system as well as a neoliberal model of citizenship which determines individual worth in terms of economic contribution.

As discussed above, an anarchist conceptualisation of mutual aid necessitates independence from state institutions and actors, because of its inherent anti-statism and opposition to power and authority. However, our data showed a tension between reconciling this central tenet of mutual aid with the imperative to deliver support in the most efficient way possible. For example, some participants collaborated with their local council because it gave their groups' activities "a validity" (Mandy, 49, Scotland) and other groups invited local police officers or councillors to their organisational meetings. Other CMAGs were ideologically opposed to collaboration with these state authorities and so chose to maintain their independence from them. These differences reflect disagreement about the purpose and nature of mutual aid (radical/charity-model) among CMAGs (see Mould et al., 2022, for a useful delineation of three different types of mutual aid).

Avoiding Politics

A further tension was identified in participants' talk about their groups – that between practicing a political and critical form of mutual aid, on the one hand, and the need to prioritise inclusivity in the group. Specifically, while many participants had strong political beliefs and opinions (e.g., on the UK government's handling of the pandemic), they tended to construct their groups as "apolitical" or not "party political" to (1) reach and attract new members of different political affiliations; and (2) reduce the likelihood of disagreements in the group and keep things "positive". The strategic management of group norms in this way, while effective, could also present difficulties:

You know, we all have our opinions on how things are going on, and particularly with all the stuff with Dominic Cummings[1] and things coming out, and you know, it's been very difficult to bite your tongue on some of these things. But we've tried to keep the group non-political so that the aims of what it's doing aren't then being diluted by arguments and negativity, and it kind of just remains positive.

(Sam, 33, West Midlands)

As discussed above, CMAGs had higher reported rates of trade union and political party membership as compared to the general UK population. Indeed, in this interview study, all participants were on the left of the ideological spectrum, and many were members of (left-wing) political parties and/or trade unions. This desire then, to keep mutual aid groups "apolitical", is notable. We explained this previously as functioning through a neoliberal lens which comprehends people as individuals "at the service of capital, divorced from the relationality of the public sphere" (O'Dwyer, Souza et al., 2022, p. 14). Aside from this, however, we note the muted radicality of a depoliticised version of mutual aid, which may have limited capacity to offer critique and offer alternatives.

What Personal Impact did Participation Have for Members?

There is now a vast body of research in social psychology which underscores the importance of social processes for health and wellbeing – the "social cure" approach. This approach supports an understanding of social identities – that part of our identities which are linked to our group memberships – as "powerful psychological resources that have an important role to play in managing and improving health" (Jetten et al., 2017, p. 789) and has applied this framework to a diverse range of physical and mental health issues, including stress, anxiety, and depression (Haslam et al., 2016), intergroup anxiety (Stevenson et al., 2020), and recovery from acquired brain injury (Muldoon et al., 2019).

A developing line of research also applies a social cure framework to understand experiences of volunteering (e.g., Bowe et al., 2020; Gray & Stevenson, 2020), which has recently been extended to the context of Covid-19 volunteering and mutual aid. Using survey data collected in the UK in June 2020, the effect of co-ordinated help-giving on wellbeing, depression, and anxiety, was positive but fully mediated by community identification and perceived sense of unity (Bowe et al., 2021). In an interview study with members of a UK mutual aid group, Mao et al. (2021) similarly found positive (e.g., positive emotional experiences, greater sense of control) and negative (stress) effects on wellbeing associated with participation in the group. Further, participants who viewed Covid-19 mutual aid in political terms reported feelings of empowerment, which was absent in the narratives of those who did not see it in this way.

Our project also set out to understand the 'social cure' of mutual aid within a political context (O'Dwyer, Beascoechea-Seguí et al., 2021). In April–May 2020, we collected survey data from 844 self-identified members of UK CMAGs or Covid-19 community response groups. Our survey contained items which tapped (1) group identification; (2) perceived support from their group; (3) perceived collective efficacy; (4) perceived group politicisation; and two measures of coping and mental health; (5) coping self-efficacy; and (6) anxiety. Following previous work (Avanzi et al., 2015; Häusser et al., 2020) we examined whether the effects of group identification on anxiety and coping self-efficacy were mediated by perceived support and perceived collective efficacy. We also tested whether these associations were moderated by perceived group politicisation.

We found support for the pathway linking group identification to coping self-efficacy via perceived support and collective efficacy, but not, contrary to previous work (Bowe et al., 2021) between group identification and anxiety. Thus, we found support for a "social cure" related to mutual aid for coping self-efficacy, but not for anxiety. This could plausibly be explained by the time of data collection, the first period of "lockdown", during which time people were experiencing perfectly normal and expected anxiety, given that we were facing an existential threat in the form of a new virus for which no vaccine was yet available. It is possible that this *collective* experience of anxiety may interact differently with social cure processes.

In line with Mao et al. (2021), we also found some support for a moderating effect of perceived group politicisation; it moderated the indirect effect of identification on coping self-efficacy via perceived support. Specifically, for those who perceived their group as more political, identification with their CMAG led to higher coping self-efficacy through perceptions of higher levels of support from their fellow group members, as compared to those who perceived their CMAGs as less political. However, correlational analyses showed that perceived group politicisation was linked to more *negative* perceptions of one's CMAG, lower identification, and lower self-reported psychological functioning.

Taken together, these findings seem slightly contradictory; perceived group politicisation seems to have an additional benefit in terms of coping self-efficacy, but the correlational results suggest that, in the main, the more a mutual aid group was perceived as political, the more negatively it was perceived and the poorer its members seemed to function psychologically. One possible response to these findings is to reflect on the relationship between political action and mental health/wellbeing in a time of crisis. What does it mean to be "well" (psychologically or physically) during a pandemic? It is a function of structural processes and societal inequalities on class, ethnicity, and other lines. Privileged social groups have been able to protect themselves whereas relatively disadvantaged groups have been much more at risk. It is possible that mutual aid groups, by exposing their members to the realities of an unequal society, could have caused them psychological distress, however it just might be that these experiences have a politicising effect (Mao et al., 2021). This could hint at a trade-off between psychological functioning or "wellness" and the solidaristic and non-hierarchical praxis linked to radical Covid-19 mutual aid. Or as Mould et al., (2022) claim, an awareness of one's vulnerability, and furthermore its sharedness, may be one possible route to resistance.

Reflections on the Politics of Covid-19 Mutual Aid

We argue here that Covid-19 mutual aid warrants a deeper interrogation in terms of its political implications. It is necessary to focus not just on the individual level outcomes of participation in these groups (i.e., for health and wellbeing), but also to look at the ways in which these groups might function politically and contribute to resistance, critique, and social change. We need to ask the question of why these groups were deemed necessary by such huge swathes at the UK population, why so many UK residents simultaneously believed that the state would not be able to provide effective support during the pandemic (O'Dwyer, Beascoechea-Seguí et al., 2022). This is a task for future research. At the same time, the media, and learned societies which support research in this field should acknowledge that Covid-19 mutual aid is not just a feel-good story about altruism and human goodness, but also an outcome of a state which has been shrunken by neo-liberal economic policies including economic austerity, over at least the past decade in the UK. These political and economic decisions ensured that Covid-19 mutual aid was necessary – it was "not a nice to have" (Tiratelli & Kaye, 2020).

We also need to look at the ways in which involvement in UK Covid-19 mutual aid might have changed political beliefs or opinions, or motivated future political action. Mao et al. (2021) suggest two processes – witnessing the difficult situations (i.e., through interacting with neighbours in extreme poverty) and perceiving the government response as inadequate – through which Covid-19 mutual aid might have a politicising effect. Other mechanisms are also possible and warrant future empirical examination. Many of the people who took part will never have been involved in volunteering or any type of community activism before, and their experiences of UK Covid-19 may have furnished them with a sense of efficacy (particularly collective efficacy). Given that previous social psychological work on collective action demonstrates the central motivating role of collective efficacy (e.g., Van Zomeren et al., 2008), what might the consequences of Covid-19 mutual aid be for future political engagement and action in the UK?

Participants also built *relationships* through their participation in CMAGs. They met and worked with their neighbours, often for the first time, some of whom were quite different to them, for example of a different class, ethnicity, age, etc. What might the implications of Covid-19 mutual aid be for intergroup relations in a divided country such as the UK, in which divisions between each of these groups are often stark, and polarisation is rife? Again, a long-term perspective on Covid-19 mutual aid is needed here to examine these sorts of questions.

To take a psychosocial view on the political implications of Covid-19 mutual aid, we must recognise that powerful "symbolic forms" or "ideology" (Thompson, 1990) provide the cultural basis for social exclusion and exploitation. From the perspective of the dominant ideology, Covid-19 mutual aid is little more than "charitable disaster relief". A new virus "emerged" from nature (unrelated to the dominant socio-economic structures), caused a pandemic that affected all social strata, and charitable altruistic individuals decided to donate some of their time and resources to mitigate the suffering of those most in need. In this narrative, the mutual aid movement amounts to a one-off relief initiative while the disaster is ongoing and is destined to disappear once the threat is over. The ethos is the unilateral provision of some resources (food, emotional support, etc.) to those who "are lacking" resources because of their "lack of adaptation" to society. It is evident that these ideological social representations are connected to what Moscovici (1976) described as the functionalist model of social influence. In this model, mutual aid as social intervention aims to enhance adaptation to reality and reinforce the social-political-economic status quo.

A critical analysis of the pandemic produces a quite different picture. Covid-19, like other zoonoses, is probably the result of the environmental catastrophe and massacre of non-human animals led by the current dominant modes of production (Paim & Alonso, 2020). Worldwide, the pandemic has caused much more morbidity and mortality among impoverished and marginalised groups and communities and may be interpreted as capitalism-driven eugenics (Preston & Firth, 2020). Covid-19 mutual aid is not individual charity, but collective solidarity and resistance to annihilation. It is not a movement solely focused on providing relief to a specific problem (Covid-19) but in fact a platform for the construction of counter-ideological social representations and practices. It does not aim at social adaptation but social transformation. What Moscovici (1976) called the genetic model of social influence is in operation here. Social change is as constant and important as social conformity.

Our research and the chapters of the present volume show that the community responses to Covid-19 provided platforms for counter-ideology including the critique of racism, classism, and sexism. In our research, participants referred to practices aiming to guarantee the human rights of underserved and ethnic minority groups, their rights to live and thrive. Female participants have been leaders of impressive Covid-19 response operations having great impact on the public sphere. The social interventions, including material and emotional support, have provided spaces where the targeted public could not only manifest their needs but also show what they had to offer. The community is not a "problem to be addressed" but an endless supply of material and psychosocial resources.

In this sense, the question if Covid-19 mutual aid "will persist" is a false question. It only makes sense if one adopts a functionalist understanding of social influence and does not consider the bottom-up processes of social transformation. From the intra-psychological, inter-personal, inter-group, and community to the societal level, these processes included the transformation of beliefs, emotions, and behaviour of individuals toward marginalised groups such as ethnic minorities, migrants, impoverished families, elderly, and disabled people; the construction of new community relationships, with bonds of support, solidarity, and friendship; the emergence of new community groups and committees; the greater influence of grassroots groups on local councils (phenomena that participants referred to in our research); the possible creation of new organisations or charities (mentioned by some of the participants that we interviewed as possible outcomes of the CMAGs); the emergence of community leaders who may influence local or national politics; the widespread diffusion of a critique of neoliberal meritocracy and individualism that may influence elections and activism; and the strengthening of social representations that challenge the state and state autocracy. The forms that the Covid-19 mutual aid phenomenon acquired will metamorphose. But, from a genetic perspective on social influence, we can see that they will certainly persist.

Acknowledgements

Many thanks to Neus Beascoechea-Seguí for her assistance with this research.

References

Avanzi, L., Schuh, S.C., Fraccaroli, F., & van Dick, R. (2015). Why does organizational identification relate to reduced employee burnout? The mediating influence of social support and collective efficacy. *Work & Stress, 29*(1), 1–10. 10.1080/02678373.2015.1004225

Andreouli, Eleni, & Brice, Emma (2021). Citizenship under COVID-19: An analysis of UK political rhetoric during the first wave of the 2020 pandemic. *Journal of Community & Applied Social Psychology, 32*, 555–572. 10.1002/casp.2526

Bowe, M., Gray, D., Stevenson, C., McNamara, N., Wakefield, J.R.H., Kellezi, B., Wilson, I., Cleveland, M., Mair, E., Halder, M., & Costa, S. (2020). A social cure in the community: A mixed-method exploration of the role of social identity in the experiences and well-being of community volunteers. *European Journal of Social Psychology, 50*(7), 1523–1539. 10.1002/ejsp.2706

Bowe, M., Wakefield, J.R.H., Kellezi, B., Stevenson, C., McNamara, N., Jones, B.A., Sumich, A., & Heym, N. (2021). The mental health benefits of community helping during crisis: Coordinated helping, community identification and sense of unity during the COVID-19 pandemic. *Journal of Community & Applied Social Psychology*, casp.2520. 10.1002/casp.2520

Carstensen, N., Mudhar, M., & Munksgaard, F.S. (2021). 'Let communities do their work': The role of mutual aid and self-help groups in the Covid-19 pandemic response. *Disasters, 45*(S1), S146–S173. 10.1111/disa.12515

Changfoot, Nadine (2007). Local Activism and Neoliberalism: Performing Neoliberal Citizenship as Resistance. Studies in Political Economy, 80, 129–14910.1080/19187 033.2007.11675087

Chevée, A. (2021). Mutual aid in north London during the Covid-19 pandemic. *Social Movement Studies*, 1–7. 10.1080/14742837.2021.1890574

Davies, B., Lalot, F., Peitz, L., Heering, M.S., Ozkececi, H., Babaian, J., Davies Hayon, K., Broadwood, J., & Abrams, D. (2021). Changes in political trust in Britain during the COVID-19 pandemic in 2020: Integrated public opinion evidence and implications. *Humanities and Social Sciences Communications*, 8(1), 1–9. 10.1057/s41599-021-00850-6

Fancourt, D., Steptoe, A., & Wright, L. (2020). The Cummings effect: Politics, trust, and behaviours during the COVID-19 pandemic. *The Lancet*, 396(10249), 464–465. 10.1016/S0140-6736(20)31690-1

Felici, M. (2020). *Social capital and the response to Covid-19*. Bennett Institute for Public Policy. https://www.bennettinstitute.cam.ac.uk/blog/social-capital-and-response-covid-19/

Gray, D., & Stevenson, C. (2020). How can 'we' help? Exploring the role of shared social identity in the experiences and benefits of volunteering. *Journal of Community & Applied Social Psychology*, 30(4), 341–353. 10.1002/casp.2448

Haslam, Catherine, Cruwys, Tegan, Haslam, S. Alexander, Dingle, Genevieve, & Chang, Melissa Xue-Ling (2016). Groups 4 Health: Evidence that a social-identity intervention that builds and strengthens social group membership improves mental health. *Journal of Affective Disorders*, 194, 188–195. 10.1016/j.jad.2016.01.010

Häusser, J.A., Junker, N.M., & van Dick, R. (2020). The how and the when of the social cure: A conceptual model of group- and individual-level mechanisms linking social identity to health and well-being. *European Journal of Social Psychology*, 50(4), 721–732. 10.1002/ejsp.2668

Jetten, J., Haslam, S.A., Cruwys, T., Greenaway, K.H., Haslam, C., & Steffens, N.K. (2017). Advancing the social identity approach to health and well-being: Progressing the social cure research agenda: Applying the social cure. *European Journal of Social Psychology*, 47(7), 789–802. 10.1002/ejsp.2333

Kadianaki, Irini, & Andreouli, Eleni (2015). Essentialism in Social Representations of Citizenship: An Analysis of Greeks' and Migrants' Discourse. *Political Psychology*, 38, 833–848. 10.1111/pops.12271

Kropotkin, P. (2017). Mutual aid: A factor of evolution. Extending Horizons Books. (Original work published in 1902).

Mak, H.W., & Fancourt, D. (2021). Predictors of engaging in voluntary work during the Covid-19 pandemic: analyses of data from 31,890 adults in the UK. *Perspectives in Public Health*. Advance online publication. 10.1177/1757913921994146

Mao, G., Drury, J., Fernandes-Jesus, M., & Ntontis, E. (2021). How participation in Covid-19 mutual aid groups affects subjective well-being and how political identity moderates these effects. *Analyses of Social Issues and Public Policy* (Early access).

Mao, G., Fernandes-Jesus, M., Ntontis, E., & Drury, J. (2020). *What have we learned so far about COVID-19 volunteering in the UK? A rapid review of the literature* [Preprint]. Public and Global Health. 10.1101/2020.11.22.20236059

Mould, O., Cole, J., Badger, A., & Brown, P. (2022). Solidarity, not charity: Learning the lessons of the Covid-19 pandemic to reconceptualise the radicality of mutual aid. *Transactions of the Institute of British Geographers*, n/a(n/a). 10.1111/tran.12553

Moscovici, S. (1976). *Social influence and social change*. Academic Press.

Muldoon, O.T., Walsh, R.S., Curtain, M., Crawley, L., & Kinsella, E.L. (2019). Social cure and social curse: Social identity resources and adjustment to acquired brain injury. *European Journal of Social Psychology*, 49(6), 1272–1282. 10.1002/ejsp.2564

O'Dwyer, E. (2020). COVID-19 mutual aid groups have the potential to increase inter-group solidarity–but can they actually do so? *British Politics and Policy at LSE*.

O'Dwyer, Emma, Souza, Luiz Gustavo Silva, & Beascoechea-Seguí, Neus (2022). Rehearsing post-Covid-19 citizenship: Social representations of UK Covid-19 mutual aid. British Journal of Social Psychology, 61, 1245–126210.1111/bjso.12535.

O'Dwyer, E., Beascoechea-Seguí, N., & Souza, L.G.S. (2021). The amplifying effect of perceived group politicization: Effects of group perceptions and identification on anxiety and coping self-efficacy among members of UK COVID-19 mutual aid groups. *Journal of Community & Applied Social Psychology, 32*(3), 423–437. 10.1002/casp.2582

Paim, C.S., & Alonso, W.J. (2020). *Pandemics, global health and consumer choices*. Cria.

Preston, J., & Firth, R. (2020). *Coronavirus, class and mutual aid in the United Kingdom*. Springer.

Rose, D.R., & Pevalin, D.J. (2003). The NS-SEC explained. In *A researcher's guide to the National Statistics Socio-Economic Classification*.

Sitrin, M., & Colectiva Sembrar (Eds.) (2020). *Pandemic Solidarity*. Pluto Press.

Spade, D. (2020). *Mutual aid: Building solidarity during this crisis (and the next)*. Verso Books.

Stevenson, C., Costa, S., Easterbrook, M.J., McNamara, N., & Kellezi, B. (2020). Social cure processes help lower intergroup anxiety among neighborhood residents. *Political Psychology, 41*(6), 1093–1111. 10.1111/pops.12667

Tiratelli, L., & Kaye, S. (2020). Communities vs coronavirus: The rise of mutual aid. *New Local Government Network*.

Thompson, J.B. (1990). *Ideology and modern culture. Critical social theory in the era of mass communication*. Polity.

van Zomeren, Martijn, Postmes, Tom, & Spears, Russell (2008). Toward an integrative social identity model of collective action: A quantitative research synthesis of three socio-psychological perspectives. Psychological Bulletin, *134*, 504–535. 10.1037/0033-2909.134.4.504

Wein, T. (2020). How mutual aid might change Britain. Retrieved July 20, 2020, from the Dignity Project, https://dignityproject.net/wp-content/uploads/2020/07/New-Solidarity-How-Mutual-Aid-might-change-Britain.pdf

Zuri, E.K. (2020, June 5). *Why we must remember the Black roots of mutual aid groups*. Gal-Dem. https://gal-dem.com/weve-been-organising-like-this-since-day-why-we-must-remember-the-black-roots-of-mutual-aid-groups/

12 Re-Constructing the Meaning of Aid through the Politicisation of Communities in a Welfare State: The Psychological Responses to the Governmental Aid Plans against Covid-19 in Turkey

S. Bengisu Akkurt, Ahmet Çoymak, and Yasin Koç

Introduction

A sudden worldwide pandemic – Covid-19 – has shown not only that the solidarity of nations against global issues is far from ideal, but also that political and economic systems in many countries have failed to build cooperation with other nations and have come up short in developing effective policies to help their citizens survive the detrimental effects of the pandemic. Therefore, the Covid-19 pandemic has caused several multi-layered crises worldwide that pose many threats to people's health, and their economic and social lives. Citizens' responses to this layered crisis seem to vary, which requires further attention from social scientists to understand the reasons behind it. For instance, trust in political and economic systems to help citizens overcome these difficulties has become an important issue in Turkey to understand people's reaction to the preventive policies and their prosocial behaviours. This reaction requires further explanation from a political psychological perspective.

Psychological studies, mostly taking only the individual-level into account, have found that people felt lonelier during the pandemic, which might have led to higher rates of anxiety, depression, sleep disorders, and emotion regulation issues (Blasco-Belled, 2022; Porter et al., 2021; Salari et al., 2020). Yet, the reasons for this were not only the feelings of isolation and loneliness due to restricted social interactions but also people's relations to the social structure. For instance, those psychological responses were found to be highly related to individuals' economic difficulties, fear of health problems and expenditures, and interruptions in education and work (Porter et al., 2021).

Recently, Thomas et al. (2022) proposed a comprehensive higher-order model of collective action: the Model of Belonging, Individual differences, Life experience and Interaction Sustaining Engagement – MOBILISE. This model explains when, why, how, and for whom, collective action manifests. Particularly, the Engagement element of the model refers to any type of action instigated by collectives of people that aims to tackle disadvantage. The model

DOI: 10.4324/9781003301905-14

encompasses micro, meso, and macro processes. Macro processes refer to the social context, including cultural, political, and economic factors such as government's performance of democracy, economic stability, and human rights. Micro and meso processes encompass group consciousness, individual differences, and collective action, as well as their interrelations. The interaction between these processes brings out a social change in society and informs us why and when collective action occurs. In this chapter, therefore, we construe mutual aid as collective action aiming to alleviate the immediate threat experienced by disadvantaged groups in Turkey during the Covid-19 pandemic. We conceptualise it through the *Engagement* aspect of this model as the enacted collective action. We also discuss why and when people participated in mutual aid, focusing on macro processes, particularly people's lack of trust in the government aid mechanism.

It is important to understand why people's responses to state aid programs have centred around the metropolitan municipalities, governed by the opposition political parties (e.g., CHP or İYİ Party). There has been a long discussion that Turkey has a strong state-centric political culture which undervalues local authorities despite strong public support for a more liberal and civic participatory democracy (for more discussion, see Keyman & İçduygu, 2005). Therefore, in the political context of Turkey, the local authorities have been situated as impartial institutions to produce programs for the residents of whole cities. These municipalities played a local, autonomous role in the eye of the public, as an impartial figure against the authoritarianism of the nation's new presidential regime. Thus, mutual aid groups, which attracted the largest public support during the pandemic, were mostly shaped around campaigns initiated by these local authorities. These campaigns challenged the government and its authority, which led the government to suppress such initiatives, which was unique to the Turkish context. In this chapter, we explain how the aid programs in Turkey have become a field of competition between the central government and the metropolitan municipalities and how reduced trust in central government led to public responses to these aid initiatives.

The Role of Political Trust in Government Aid Plans

Trust plays a crucial role in building and maintaining social cohesion and integration within a society, but it is also the result of social transformation within the modern state. This view suggests that the best place to look for a definition of trust is in the social processes and structures that support it (for more discussion, see Çoymak et al., 2015). In the midst of a global health crisis, it is critical to reconceptualise trust since not only are there diverse levels of citizens' political trust, such as institutional, government performance, and ideological, but also because social transformation and communities' reactions to the policies have shaped the *meaning* of political trust (Dal & Tokdemir, 2022).

In the event of a catastrophic occurrence, such as a health crisis, welfare states are expected to act differently from other nations because their economic systems are already intended to build the financial and social mechanisms to support citizens in despair. However, the Covid-19 pandemic demonstrates that many countries have failed to form alliances with other countries and have fallen short of developing effective policies to mitigate the detrimental effects of Covid-19. Therefore, people's trust of their government, other citizens, and citizen groups becomes crucial to understanding how they respond to the Covid-19 pandemic, why they build mutual aid mechanisms, who they help, and in what ways they mobilise against the government's failed policies against the pandemic. A significant proportion of these questions can be explained from a political psychological perspective. Thus, in this chapter, we also use Thomas and McGarty's (2017) support model (e.g., *benevolent support* vs. *activist support*) to better understand motivations for engaging in mutual aid groups. We contend that people have mobilised through mutual aid groups not only because of a lack of support from the government but also because of decreased political trust. We argue that one reason for this was that people perceived the government's aid policies as hierarchical, dishonest, and exclusionary, especially in those communities that are not valued by the conservative norms of the government.

Citizen Expectations vs. Insufficiency of Assistance in the Welfare State: Lack of Governmental Responses to the Pandemic

The pandemic has exposed and increased existing income inequality in societies around the world (Aspachs et al., 2021; Deaton, 2021). Those of lower socioeconomic status and from disadvantaged social groups have been more likely to suffer from job loss, a decline in household income, and food insecurity (Milovanska-Farrington, 2021; Singh et al., 2021). A wide range of sectors worldwide, including agriculture, health services, transportation, tourism, and sports, were forced to reduce or pause their activities and suffered massive financial losses (Olufadewa et al., 2021). Turkey was not exempt from this trend. Just a month after the first Covid-19 case was reported on 10 March 2020, Turkey was among the top 10 countries with the highest number of Covid-19 cases (Çakır, 2020). Although a full lockdown on industry and business during workdays was never introduced, the pandemic was enough to exacerbate the economic depression in Turkey, where people were already struggling with the country's economic downturn (Açikgöz & Günay, 2020).

As of 2018, the Turkish lira began to lose value rapidly; there were sudden fluctuations in exchange rates, inflation, and foreign currency debt (World Bank, 2021). According to economists, the most important reasons for these were the rising authoritarian approach after transferring from a parliamentary to presidential political system in the country and the ensuing policies which did not comply with the recommendations of most economists in the financial interest policy (Daragahi, 2018), such as not raising interest rates as required by the market. The World Bank's report also showed that the decrease in overall purchasing power was felt intensely in Turkey, especially among low-income households. During this period, the global media covered a lot of news about the depreciation of the Turkish lira, the people crushed by debt, and falling purchasing power (Sarı, 2020; Soner, 2021). Due to the Turkish economy's ongoing decline, the state aid plans were often insufficient, even in sectors where the government focused its financial support, such as health care.

İpek and Acar's (2022) comparative analysis of six countries, including Turkey, shows that the lack of transparency and legal infrastructure has had a significant negative impact on budget performance during the Covid-19-related economic recession. Therefore, Turkey's income loss, unemployment, and bankruptcy level are at the highest of all time. Especially small businesses were among the groups hardest hit by the pandemic, with approximately 125,000 going bankrupt within the first year of the pandemic (Süzer, 2021).

Public expectations of state support in a welfare state are higher than those of other countries with different political systems (Daly & Lewis, 2000) because these states have tax revenues to balance income inequality by providing the necessary social and financial support for their citizens. Although Turkey has specific tax items for natural disasters, including health crises, soon after the outbreak of the pandemic, people's expectations were disappointed and trust in the government decreased to a certain extent. The presidential approval rate as of July 2021 was the lowest in six years according to the Metropol Turkey Pulse (Metropoll, 2021). Therefore, it is not surprising to see the figure that the government spent only 7.2% of Turkey's GDP on Covid-19 expenditures, including all economic, health, and social aid schemes (DİSK-AR, 2021) as compared to 12% in France, 18% in the UK and 20% in Australia.

Two significant events, among many others, have had a strong impact on reducing the public expectation of the governmental performance during the pandemic. First, the government shared an international bank account number (IBAN) with the public to increase income for the support program. It is common for civic societies and voluntary organisations to ask for money by sharing IBAN publicly to increase revenue for causes. Yet, the state that was supposed to protect its citizens acted as if it was a non-governmental organisation. Therefore, sharing IBAN with the public was perceived as proof of the economy's downfall as opposed to common discourses of the government regarding the strong Turkish economy. The second event was a tourism campaign video, released on May 13, 2020 – "GoTürkiye" – which the Culture and Tourism Ministry shared to urge tourists to come to Turkey and spend *a safe holiday*. In the campaign video, tourism staff are featured wearing yellow masks printed with "Enjoy – I am vaccinated", simulating a smiling emoji. Although the ministry immediately removed the video after a strong public reaction, it was another sign in the eyes of the public that the authoritarian neoliberal policies of the Turkish government were rather inadequate to build effective financial aid responses for helping its citizens, as the government was concerned about attracting tourism while most of its own citizens were unvaccinated (Atalay, 2022).

Since the beginning of the pandemic, one of the areas that government support has prioritised the most has been health services. For instance, five days after the first case was seen on March 15, all private hospitals were declared pandemic hospitals, and those without health insurance were assured of free treatment for Covid-19. However, the government's failure to effectively implement a suppression plan and the early withdrawal of pandemic restrictions due to economic pressures led to an increase in the number of cases. There have been periods when some patients were not admitted to intensive care units because hospital capacity was exceeded (Öztürk, 2020). Furthermore, the Ministry of Health's lack of transparency in data sharing because of the strong desire of the government to consolidate its political power during the economic downturn resulted in inconsistencies across public institutions, making it unable to develop effective and timely health policies (Mardin, 2021). Also, the government's aid programs for public engagement to preventive measures failed operationally, leading people to question the performance of the government's aid plans. For instance, the government's weekly five free masks initiative for citizens aged between 20 and 65 (full lockdown imposed for the rest of the citizens) via the PTT (Post and Telegraph Organisation) failed due to resource limits and organisational disruptions in the supply of masks (Hoşbaş, 2020).

Several economic and social support packages developed by the government during the pandemic were also questioned. The government declared the first economic support package as covering broader concerns about the economy but did not provide a detailed action plan. The package mostly focused on helping large companies, financial actors, and big industries. The only items in this package were two billion TL (£260k) of economic support, corresponding to families in need and people who lost income (Karakış, 2020). Even the aid item for those who lost income was introduced with a restrictive condition that the workplace should be partially or fully closed for more than four weeks. The amount of support was calculated at 60% of the insured's average daily gross wage. Therefore, a rough estimation suggests that only three and a half million out of 27 million employees in Turkey benefited from this aid for three months. According to a recent report (DISK-AR, 2021), citizens benefited from only 22% of the whole governmental aid schemes, while the rest was spent on protecting businesses. Therefore, the governmental aid plans were criticised not only because of their insufficiency but also because of their lack of transparency in explaining the source of the money to cover the announced economic package. Moreover, people were angry at tax reductions for big companies, the tourism industry, and the encouragement of airline transportation to support airline companies at a time when people were encouraged to stay at home and blamed the government for not focusing on necessary aid structures like employment support (Demiralp, 2020).

The Context of the State's Exclusionary Aid Programmes: The Dynamics of Politicisation and Polarisation

Overall, the economic support was insufficient even for the groups and sectors that received the most economic assistance from the state. The indicators of the Turkish economy and the experiences of citizens and local business owners highlighted the inadequacy of the government's pandemic aid in public opinion.

The budget allocated for aid was very low, considering the country's poverty line and minimum subsistence level. Moreover, the government's pandemic assistance was primarily directed toward large economic entities in the production, industry, tourism, and food and beverage industries. However, other corporate sectors, particularly those that were not considered compatible with the government's conservative principles, felt, on the other hand, that they were purposefully excluded from the state's economic assistance. Artists, entertainment sector workers such as musicians and theatre staff, businesses selling alcohol, and small shopkeepers were among those groups that thought they benefited the least from pandemic economic support (Karaoglan, 2021).

Furthermore, the pandemic hit the cinema industry, entertainment venue operators, and alcohol-selling venue owners the hardest (Hurtas, 2021; Yazıcıoğlu & Karabulut, 2021). Owners of liquor stores and entertainment venues that served alcoholic beverages, as well as those who worked there, felt particularly excluded because the restrictions for these venues remained in place even after the lockdown was lifted from the coffee shops and restaurants serving only soft drinks (Yazıcıoğlu & Karabulut, 2021).

Another public controversy surrounding the government health-related restrictions was that the live music, festival, and concert ban after midnight remained in effect even after the lockdown. These limitations were heavily criticised by the entertainment venue businesses and musicians (Çelik & Özer, 2021). Therefore, the public has questioned whether the government's intention behind restrictions was to to support citizens and prioritise public health during the pandemic or to exert more control over those politically different groups. Indeed, critics of the government have claimed that its restriction plans and aid schemes were targeted to exclude communities with secular lifestyles or that opposed the government's conservative principles (Hurtas, 2021).

Individuals formed mutual aid groups in their communities to help their neighbours and fellow citizens survive the pandemic's detrimental effects and the failure of the governmental effort. In this political context, metropolitan municipalities came up with non-partisan inclusive aid schemes to attract mutual aid groups engaging in these efforts. An organic political relation has been formed across the mutual aid groups, concentrated around the municipality aid initiatives that challenged the government's powerful image. Consequently, the central government attempted to prevent or hinder these activities. As a result, people have become more politicised through the mutual aid groups by supporting and actively engaging in municipalities' pandemic response efforts.

Public Responses to Government Aid in Turkey: Change in Exclusionary Governmental Aid towards the Emergence of Mutual Aid Groups

Collective action is goal-oriented, aiming to improve the conditions of a group (Wright et al., 1990). So far, collective action has been examined in psychology by extensively focusing on meso level predictors, such as group consciousness. Group consciousness constitutes membership of a group (e.g., social identification), group efficacy (e.g., believing that the group can change things), and injustice (e.g., believing that your group is worse off than others). These elements work together to lead to collective action (van Zomeren et al., 2008). However, group consciousness does not by itself explain collective action, and all these predictors combined do not incorporate macro-level contextual elements. A number of other factors, such as individual differences (e.g., morality and ideology) and life experiences (e.g., intergroup contact, injustice perceptions), also shape group consciousness (Duncan, 2018; Thomas et al., 2022). They help explain when people collectivise their individual disadvantage experiences and why and how they decide to act against it instead of disengaging or not acting. Therefore, to understand why people have mobilised through mutual aid groups in Turkey, we need to analyse the macro-level political context as well as how benevolent support schemes of the government affects group consciousness in this political context.

Mutual aid refers to the voluntary exchange of resources for mutual benefit, such as financial aid, food aid, health and hygiene products, and any other assistance required in times of distress. Therefore, a mutual aid group can be described as ordinary people banding together to help each other, cooperating, understanding, and showing solidarity, realising that the established governmental and non-governmental structures cannot meet their needs; the difference from a charity is significant in this regard (Izlar, n.d.). While some researchers consider mutual aid as a type of immediate crisis response, others believe that mutual aid groups have the potential to cause more radical positive changes in social structures (O'Dwyer et al., 2022). The reason to expect the potential for change in the structure through mutual aid groups could be the politicisation of an individual that the political system and social structure have become more visible for the individual through experiences of sharing various disadvantages with other citizen groups. The Turkish case could be an example of this. During the pandemic in Turkey, the economic support expected from the state and the government's preventive measures were not only insufficient in many respects but also discriminatory towards some citizen groups, which paved the way for the emergence of various mutual aid groups to compensate for these deficiencies. The mutual aid groups attracted a large number of citizens. However, uniquely in the history of Turkey, these groups were gathered around the initiatives of the metropolitan municipalities of Istanbul and Ankara governed by the opposition political party that may show the politicisation of individuals towards a more inclusive political system.

In Turkey, like in other welfare states, the public expected the government to respond effectively to protect all citizens from the negative effects of the pandemic. However, giving priority to sustaining the economic welfare of large companies, financial actors, and big industries and failing to develop inclusive and sufficient aid mechanisms for the public has shaken people's trust in the state and raised uncertainties about how to overcome health crises in various communities in Turkey (Çakır, 2020; Dal & Tokdemir, 2022). Therefore, people were looking for a new way to build solidarity with their fellow citizens in fighting against the negative effects of the pandemic. Aid campaigns offered by metropolitan municipalities in Turkey provided an outlet for this.

Municipality-initiated aid mechanisms differed from government-initiated aid mechanisms in some respects. While the state's aid policies were almost entirely focused on benevolent aid such as cash assistance and tax relief, community support campaigns of the metropolitan municipalities have integrated more activist forms of aid into their campaigns along with some benevolent aid. For instance, although the municipalities provided aid that would fall under benevolent support, such as financial assistance, food assistance, and rent assistance, they prioritised activist support by establishing various campaigns. These campaigns enabled the formation of new mutual aid groups in local communities, but also helped to increase the size of mutual aid groups and matched volunteers with those in need (OECD, 2020). People perceived these activities as impartial, inclusive, and encouraging autonomy and sustainability. Those might be the significant reasons why they received massive public support as we know anecdotally which could be further investigated using archival data.

The Istanbul Municipality's *Askıda Ekmek* [Hanging Bread] campaign is an example of an activist support action led by a metropolitan municipality. In this campaign, people could pay for extra loaves of bread at their local bakery and those in need could take these loaves for free. This easily mobilised people to form or engage with a mutual aid group in their community. The public's enthusiasm for this campaign encouraged other municipalities to launch various similar campaigns. Afterwards, Istanbul and Ankara municipalities set up an online system to match volunteers with those who could not pay their electricity, water, and heating bills, namely *Askıda Fatura* [Hanging Bills] and *Ankara Tek Yürek* (n.d.) [Ankara One Heart] campaigns. Public support for these campaigns was even bigger than the previous one because, unlike most governmental aid, metropolitan campaigns paid more attention to the public's basic needs and demands, provided more concrete solutions to specific issues, were more transparent and solidarity-based, and less hierarchical in the sense that people helped each other rather than were given help from top-down.

The government, however, was not pleased by the public support for the municipalities' aid initiatives and took steps to hinder these activities, which had the opposite effect and increased public support for the municipalities' aid campaigns. For example, the government prevented municipalities from increasing the number of kiosks, which are symbols of the *Askıda Ekmek* campaign and where Istanbul municipality sells bread at a lower price than the market, and where the donated bread of mutual aid groups was delivered to those who needed it. The campaign received 6.2 million TL in public donations. However, the government confiscated the donated money through legislation and forced its transfer to the government's financial office. The government tried to legitimise the confiscation of public donations by emphasising that the state should be the only official body to look after any public donations and prevent any possible wrongdoing with them. However, the municipalities run by the government party continued collecting donations without any difficulties. Moreover, the implication that the local municipalities and people supporting them were untrustworthy mobilised even more people to support metropolitan municipalities' aid campaigns. Therefore, the mutual aid groups expanded with more sustainable support and engagement of citizens.

Several campaigns by these municipalities provided a space for people to form or join a mutual aid group. Providing a venue for musicians and orchestra artists who had no income during the pandemic to perform their art, setting up a web page for online theatre performances, and offering free stage opportunities to cinemas and independent artists were not all but a few of them. Mutual aid groups like *Istanbul Volunteers* developed from these municipal campaigns and organised free workshops, events, and training to help with various psychosocial issues that arose during the lockdown.

In conclusion, we know in most cases *why* people engage in collective action (e.g., motivation) to restore justice in their local community (Della Porta & Tarrow, 2005), yet it is still unknown *when* people will engage (Livingstone, 2014). In the context of mutual aid in Turkey, structural reasons such as a lack of governmental support, perceived injustice, and low governmental trust could explain why people mobilised to engage with mutual aid groups. However, it would not be wrong to claim from a political psychological perspective that the activist aid campaigns of these metropolitan municipalities where government assistance was less focused, and discriminatory, were a turning point to mobilise the public to engage with mutual aid groups.

References

Açikgöz, Ö., & Günay, A. (2020). The early impact of the Covid-19 pandemic on the global and Turkish economy. *Turkish Journal of Medical Sciences*, *50*(SI-1), 520–526. 10.3906/sag-2004-6

Ankara Tek Yürek (n.d.) Ankara Büyükşehir Belediyesi. https://www.ankaratekyurek.com/

Aspachs, O., Durante, R., Graziano, A., Mestres, J., Reynal-Querol, M., & Montalvo, J.G. (2021). Tracking the impact of Covid-19 on economic inequality at high frequency. *PLOS One*, *16*(3). 10.1371/journal.pone.0249121

Atalay, S. (2022). 'The ones who die are lost and the survivors are what we have': Neoliberal governmentality and the governance of Covid-19 risk in social media posts in Turkey. *Health, Risk & Society*, *24*, 1–22. 10.1080/13698575.2022.2056583

Blasco-Belled, A., Tejada-Gallardo, C., Fatsini-Prats, M., & Alsinet, C. (2022). Mental health among the general population and healthcare workers during the Covid-19 pandemic: A meta-analysis of well-being and psychological distress prevalence. *Current Psychology*. 10.1007/s12144-022-02913-6

Çakır, B. (2020). Covid-19 in Turkey: Lessons learned. *Journal of Epidemiology and Global Health*, *10*(2), 115–117. 10.2991/jegh.k.200520.001

Çelik, G. & Özer, T. (2021, March 5). Alkollü işletmeler: Salgın bahane edildi, olan bize oldu. *Cumhuriyet.* https://www.cumhuriyet.com.tr/haber/alkollu-isletmeler-salgin-bahane-edildi-olan-bize-oldu-1818398

Çoymak, A., Gheorghiu, M., Niens, U., & Lyons, E. (2015). Vatandaşlığın Psikolojisi ve Politik Güven. *Siyaset Psikolojisi*, *1*, 229–242. 10.13140/RG.2.1.3104.3682

Dal, A., & Tokdemir, E. (2022). Social-psychology of vaccine intentions: The mediating role of institutional trust in the fight against Covid-19. *Political Behavior*, *44*, 1459–1481. 10.1007/s11109-022-09793-3

Daly, M., & Lewis, J. (2000) The concept of social care and the analysis of contemporary welfare states. *British Journal of Sociology*, *51*(2), 281–298. 10.1111/j.1468-4446.2000.00281.x

Daragahi, B. (2018, May 25). Erdogan is failing economics 101. *Foreign Policy.* https://foreignpolicy.com/2018/05/25/erdogan-is-a-mad-economist-and-turkey-is-his-laboratory/

Deaton, A. (2021). Covid-19 and global income inequality. *LSE Public Policy Review*, *1*(4). 10.31389/lseppr.26

Della Porta, D., & Tarrow, S. (2005). Transnational protest and global activism: People, passions. In A.F. Blackwell & D. MacKay (Eds.), *Power*. Cambridge University Press.

Demiralp, S. (2020, March 19). Koronavirüs ekonomik tedbir paketi: Kime, hangi güvence sunuluyor? *BBC.* https://www.bbc.com/turkce/haberler-dunya-51958762

DİSK-AR (2021). Dünyada ve Türkiye'de Covid-19'un sosyal ve ekonomik etkileri için ayrılan kaynaklar (2). *DİSK.* http://disk.org.tr/2021/08/disk-ardan-yeni-rapor-salgin-azami-destek-asgari/

Duncan, L.E. (2018). The psychology of collective action. In K. Deaux & M. Snyder (Eds.), *The Oxford handbook of personality and social psychology* (2nd edition, pp. 885–907). Oxford University Press.

Hoşbaş, T. (2020, May 4). Bilecik'te gönüllü kursiyerlerden maske üretim seferberliğine destek. *AA.* https://www.aa.com.tr/tr/yasam/bilecikte-gonullu-kursiyerlerden-maske-uretim-seferberligine-destek/1828132

Hurtas, S. (2021). Critics say Erdogan used pandemic to kill Turkey's nightlife. *Al-Monitor.* https://www.al-monitor.com/originals/2021/06/critics-say-erdogan-used-pandemic-kill-turkeys-nightlife#ixzz7Ql7prOjn

İpek, E. A. Ş., & Acar, İ. A. (2022). Covid-19 outbreak and budget management: An assessment for Turkey within the framework of selected country examples. In Açıkgöz, B . & Acar, I. A.. (Eds.), *Pandemnomics: The pandemic's lasting economic effects* (pp. 151–184). Singapore: Springer.

Izlar, J. (n.d.) *What is mutual aid?* School of Social Work University of Georgia. Retrieved April 9, 2020, from https://ssw.uga.edu/news/article/what-is-mutual-aid-by-joel-izlar/

Karakış, G. (2020, March 19). 100 milyar TL'lik kalkan. *Hürriyet.* https://www.hurriyet.com.tr/ekonomi/100-milyar-tllik-kalkan-41472244

Karaoglan, S. (2021). The challenges of the Turkish music-entertainment industry during the Covid-19 pandemic. In *Contemporary Issues with Multidisciplinary Perspectives on Social Science* (pp. 305–316). Peter Lang.

Keyman, E.F., & İçduygu, A. (2005). Citizenship, identity, and the question of democracy in Turkey. In Keyman, E.F. & İçduygu, A. (Eds.), *Citizenship in a global world European questions and Turkish experiences* (pp. 1–27). Routledge.

Livingstone, A.G. (2014). Why the psychology of collective action requires qualitative transformation as well as quantitative change. *Contemporary Social Science*, *9*(1), 121–134. 10.1080/21582041.2013.851404

Mardin, F.D. (2021). Turkey's healthcare policies and the Covid-19 pandemic. In Balcı, B., Bourmaud, P., & Kaya, S. (Eds.), *Analyses pluridisciplinaires sur la crise sanitaire Covid-19 en Turquie*. Istanbul: Institut français d'études anatoliennes. 10.4000/books.ifeagd.3774

Metropoll (2021). *Türkiye'nin Nabzı – Nisan 2021*. Metropoll Stratejik Araştırmalar. http://www.metropoll.com.tr/arastirmalar/turkiyenin-nabzi-17/1898

Milovanska-Farrington, S. (2021). Job loss and food insecurity during the Covid-19 pandemic. *Journal of Economic Studies*. 10.2139/ssrn.3823640

O'Dwyer, E., Souza, L.G.S., & Beascoechea-Seguí, N. (2022). Rehearsing post-Covid-19 citizenship: Social representations of UK Covid-19 mutual aid. *British Journal of Social Psychology*, *61*, 1245–1262. Advance online publication. 10.1111/bjso.12535

OECD (2020). *OECD policy responses to coronavirus (Covid-19): Cities policy responses*. OECD. https://www.oecd.org/coronavirus/policy-responses/cities-policy-responses-fd1053ff/#section-d1e399

Olufadewa, I.I., Adesina, M.A., Oladele, R.I., Oladoye, M.J., Akinmuleya, T., & Ogunleye, E. (2021). COVID-19 and the economy: Job loss and economic shutdown. *Medical Research Journal*, *6*(2), 125–130. 10.5603/mrj.a2021.0019

Öztürk, F. (2020, November). Koronavirüs: Doktorlar 'Covid-19 yoğun bakım yatakları doldu, servislerde yer kalmadı' uyarısı yapıyor. *BBC*. https://www.bbc.com/turkce/haberler-turkiye-54935115

Porter, C., Favara, M., Hittmeyer, A., Scott, D., Sánchez Jiménez, A., Ellanki, R., Woldehanna, T., Duc, L.T., Craske, M.G., & Stein, A. (2021). Impact of the Covid-19 pandemic on anxiety and depression symptoms of young people in the global south: Evidence from a four-country cohort study. *BMJ Open*, *11*(4), e049653. 10.1101/2021.02.02.21250897

Salari, N., Hosseinian-Far, A., Jalali, R., Vaisi-Raygani, A.S., Mohammadi, M.S., & Khaledi-Paveh, B. (2020). Prevalence of stress, anxiety, depression among the general population during the Covid-19 pandemic: A systematic review and meta-analysis. *Globalisation and Health*, *16*. https://doi.org/0.1186/s12992-020-00589-w

Sarı, D. (2020, July 23). Pandemi borç alevini büyütüyor. *Bloomberg HT*. https://www.bloomberght.com/pandemi-borc-alevini-buyutuyor-2260684

Singh, K., Kondal, D., Mohan, S., Jaganathan, S., Deepa, M., Venkateshmurthy, N.S., Jarhyan, P., Anjana, R.M., Narayan, K.M.V., Mohan, V., Tandon, N., Ali, M.K., Prabhakaran, D., & Eggleston, K. (2021). Health, psychosocial, and economic impacts of the Covid-19 pandemic on people with chronic conditions in India: A mixed methods study. *BMC Public Health*, *21*(1). 10.1186/s12889-021-10708-w

Soner, S. (2021, Nov 21). Türk Lirası eriyor, vatandaşın alım gücü günden güne düşüyor. *T24*. https://t24.com.tr/haber/turk-lirasi-eriyor-vatandasin-alim-gucu-gunden-gune-dusuyor-belirsizlikten-sikayetci-esnaf-ve-tuccar-gelismeleri-degerlendirdi-kimse-mutlu-degil-zarar-etmezsek-seviniyoruz,995737

Süzer, E. (2021, April 4). 125 bin esnaf iflas bayrağını çekti. *Sözcü*. https://www.sozcu.com.tr/2021/ekonomi/125-bin-esnaf-iflas-bayragini-cekti-6352763/

Thomas, E.F., Duncan, L., McGarty, C., Louis, W.R., & Smith, L.G.E. (2022). MOBI-LISE: A higher-order integration of collective action research to address global challenges. *Advances in Political Psychology*. Advance online publication. 10.1111/pops.12811

Thomas, E.F., & McGarty, C. (2017). Giving versus acting: Using latent profile analysis to distinguish between benevolent and activist support for global poverty reduction. *British Journal of Social Psychology*, *57*(1), 189–209. 10.1111/bjso.12228

Van Zomeren, M., Postmes, T., & Spears, R. (2008). Toward an integrative social identity model of collective action: A quantitative research synthesis of three socio-psychological perspectives. *Psychological Bulletin*, *134*(4), 504–535. 10.1037/0033-2909.134.4.504

World Bank. (2021). *Turkey economic monitor, April 2021: Navigating the waves*. World Bank. https://openknowledge.worldbank.org/handle/10986/35497

Wright, S.C., Taylor, D.M., & Moghaddam, F.M. (1990). The relationship of perceptions and emotions to behavior in the face of collective inequality. *Social Justice Research*, *4*(3), 229–250. 10.1007/bf01048399

Yazıcıoğlu, Y. & Karabulut, M. (2021, November 12). Beş Soru Beş Yanıtta Corona Virüs Salgınında Son Durum. *Amerikanın Sesi*. https://www.amerikaninsesi.com/a/bes-soru-bes-yanitta-corona-virusu-salgininda-son-durum/6310584.html

13 Covid-19, Carnival, and Community in New Orleans, 2020

Martha Radice

Introduction

New Orleans, Louisiana, was hit hard by Covid-19 in March 2020. The parades and parties of carnival season, which had culminated on Mardi Gras Day, 25 February in 2020, were instrumental in its spread. Yet carnival was also the source of many community initiatives to mitigate the negative material, social, and psychological effects of the pandemic. Drawing on the ethnographic research I have been conducting since 2016, this chapter analyses how the voluntary social clubs that produce carnival, called "krewes", responded to the first four months of the pandemic, with a focus on "new-wave" krewes (a term I explain below). First, I outline my research and the initial spread and impact of Covid-19 in New Orleans. I then discuss the projects of creativity, sociability, and solidarity that new-wave carnival krewes undertook. I conclude by arguing that the social relations of carnival not only provided the foundation for relief initiatives, but also the motivation to tackle the pandemic at a collective level.

Researching Carnival in New Orleans

My ethnographic research explores the practices of new-wave carnival krewes in New Orleans. A "krewe" is a social club that organizes events during carnival season, which runs from Twelfth Night (6 January) to Mardi Gras (Fat Tuesday), 47 days before Easter Sunday. These events are typically a public parade and a private ball, although some krewes hold only one or the other. The hundreds of carnival krewes vary in longevity, degree of formal organization, gender and racial composition, social class, politics, and aesthetics. One key distinction is whether their parade has members riding floats pulled by tractors or walking alongside floats pulled by mules, bicycles, or humans. Most large float parades roll uptown, along broad Saint Charles Avenue, while the smaller-scale krewes parade along narrower streets in neighbourhoods downriver of Canal Street, so they are sometimes called "downtown" carnival krewes (Wade et al., 2019). Their politics tend to be progressive and satirical, and their costumes, throws, and floats are usually made by members, not

DOI: 10.4324/9781003301905-15

professionals or manufacturers. ("Throws" are trinkets, often beads, that paraders throw to spectators, making carnival parades especially interactive.) I call these krewes "new-wave", in contrast to elite "old-line" or other mainstream krewes. They emerged from the counter-cultural movements of the 1960s–1970s and have proliferated in the 15 years since Hurricane Katrina, yet their scale and ethos hark back to the free-form street carnival of the early 19th century, before the first float parade appeared in 1857 (Gill, 1997).

New-wave krewes are only one element of carnival, which is a complex, lively field of cultural production (Kinser, 1990). Reflecting New Orleans society, carnival is socially stratified and relatively racially segregated. New-wave krewes tend to be made up of mostly white, college-educated middle-class people. Of similar composition and vintage are the troupes of women or men who dance or otherwise perform between floats in uptown parades (a few of which I mention below). African American traditions include the Mardi Gras Indians or Black Masking Indians (Becker, 2013; Fi Yi Yi et al., 2018; Lipsitz, 1988), Baby Dolls (Vaz, 2013), and Zulu Social Aid and Pleasure Club (Smith, 2013). Gay carnival krewes stage spectacular *tableaux vivants* at balls, like extravagantly costumed fashion shows, rather than parading (Smith, 2017; Wolff, 2011). There is a suburban tradition of "truck parades", in which families, friends, and neighbours decorate and ride on flatbed trucks (Roberts, 2006). Many individuals participate in more than one kind of carnival group, while others just celebrate at home or in the streets with friends, family, and strangers. Carnival is also influenced by other local cultural practices, like second line parades (Regis 1999).

I have conducted 13 months of ethnographic fieldwork, mainly participant observation and semi-structured interviews, in New Orleans over six years. The material for this chapter, however, was gathered remotely. Social media, primarily Facebook, was already one way I keep up with people, events, and conversations in the field (cf. Dalsgaard, 2016). It became even more important when Covid-19 cut short a planned six-month fieldwork trip in March 2020 (Radice, 2020). I followed how the pandemic unfolded in New Orleans through social media and online newspaper, magazine, radio, and TV reports. I kept in touch with friends and conducted interviews by phone and on video-conferencing platforms. Like Horst and Miller (2012), I maintain that the so-called virtual world of social media is not separate from some "real" world but can only be understood in relation to the non-digital social milieus in which it is embedded. My digital ethnography would make little sense without my in-person ethnography. I do take extra care over the ethics of digital ethnography, since social media are a complex amalgam of public and private (Willis, 2019). Here, I only discuss social media material from public posts, though these might have reached me through private re-shares.

Covid-19 in New Orleans

New Orleans was an early "hotspot" of Covid-19 in the USA. Its first case was confirmed on 9 March, 14 days after Mardi Gras. The outbreak spiralled from

74 cases and two confirmed deaths by 15 March to 1834 cases and 101 deaths by 31 March. When New Orleans' per capita Covid-19 death rate outstripped New York City's at the end of March, national media outlets began to blame carnival for the spread of the disease and Mayor LaToya Cantrell for not cancelling it, though no other American cities were restricting large gatherings at that time (Radice, 2020). It transpired that the parades and parties of carnival 2020 had indeed been super-spreading events (Zeller et al., 2021), but many New Orleanians resisted the carnival-shaming narrative. They countered that it was not carnival but the city's entrenched social inequality — its dependence on tourism and service-sector jobs with low wages and inadequate benefits, systemic racism, unaffordable/overcrowded housing, and privatised, in-accessible healthcare—that made it structurally vulnerable to the Covid-19 pandemic (Adams & Johnson, 2020; Losh & Plyer, 2020). The impact of Covid-19 was uneven, however. Infection and death rates were much higher among African Americans, who make up 60% of the New Orleans population, than whites, likely because African Americans were more likely than whites to live in multigenerational households and work in essential frontline jobs like retail and healthcare (Weinstein & Plyer, 2020).

With support from Louisiana Governor John Bel Edwards (a Democrat), Mayor Cantrell implemented a mandate to "Stay at Home" except for es-sential activities on 20 March. The rolling seven-day average of new cases in New Orleans peaked on April 7 at 444, then dropped off quickly and did not exceed 150 from 14 April until 3 December (City of New Orleans Covid-19 data dashboard, accessed via https://ready.nola.gov/incident/coronavirus/ on April 1, 2022). Phase One of a four-phase reopening plan began on 15 May. It allowed gatherings of a "household size," asked people to limit their contacts to "a small and consistent 'crew,'" and mandated masks or face coverings for activities in public (except outdoor, distanced recreation). On 13 June, Phase Two began, which retained masking and distancing guidelines but permitted indoor gatherings of up to 25 people and outdoor gatherings of 50, and reopened many businesses and public places at reduced capacity. At first, bars reopened, but a resurgence of infections led to their closure in late July. New Orleans did not move to Phase Three of reopening until October 2020. Most activities I discuss in this chapter took place under the Stay Home Order and Phase One, during which time carnival networks proved to be a source of diversion, comfort, and succour.

Creativity

New-wave carnival krewes combined their skills in costuming with digital technologies and social media to make creative entertainment. New Orleans' public culture features many parades outside of carnival season; indeed, the first events that Mayor Cantrell cancelled were second line parades scheduled for 15 March, Saint Patrick's Day parades (17 March), and the Mardi Gras Indian parades held around Saint Joseph's Day (19 March). Some new-wave krewes that were due to parade in April created virtual alternatives. The Krewe du Fool replaced their April Fool's Day parade with a 5-minute compilation of images of members in their costumes, framed with comical scenes of an impatient spectator (Krewe Du Fool, 2020). The Flaming Flagettes, a "drag flag dancing troupe" who would have participated in the Gay Easter Parade on 12 April, made a sophisticated six-and-a-half-minute parody of the newly popular videoconferencing platform Zoom (Page, 2020, and see Clapp, 2020). Twelve Flagettes appear in their little squares, mostly in "speaker view" mode but sometimes in "gallery view" and occasionally upside-down. They wake up, put on colourful wigs, make-up and costume, dance and lip-sync to a pop medley, waving tiny replicas of their signature flame flags. Their finale is, appropriately, Whitney Houston's "I wanna dance with somebody".

New-wave carnival krewes also embraced the viral video phenomenon known as the #dontrushchallenge, after the soundtrack of the first version, or the #(passthe)brushchallenge. Each #brushchallenge video begins with a person wearing ordinary clothes doing an everyday activity at home. They catch an object thrown to them from off-camera, often a make-up brush (hence the name), which they brush against the camera lens. This creates a moment of darkness from which they magically emerge looking entirely different, in costume, regalia, or glamorous clothes. They strike a pose, then throw their brush in the same direction to the next person (so if they caught it from above, they drop it below). *Teen Vogue* reports that this trend was started by eight students, all women of colour, who were locked down in their university residences (Isama, 2020). The challenge became particularly popular among Black and Indigenous women celebrating their collective strength and beauty, while other versions came from costuming specialists like cosplay fans and gender-non-conforming make-up artistes. It was a way for groups centred on shared identity, ethnicity, hobby, or friendship to showcase their aesthetic and come together while apart.

A dozen new-wave carnival krewes challenged each other to create #passthebrushchallenge videos.[1] They usually used a krewe-specific throw as their transition object, and the "everyday" segments sometimes related to the krewe's theme. For instance, some of the Rolling Elvi – men who dress as Elvis Presley and ride motor scooters in several uptown parades – are polishing Elvis memorabilia or looking at Elvis records before they catch the krewe-branded poker chip and turn into their version of the man himself, to a soundtrack, naturally, of Elvis (Krewe of the Rolling Elvi, 2020).

The Krewe of Krampus made a particularly involved #passthebrushchallenge video (Krewe of Krampus New Orleans, 2020). This krewe, founded in 2015, parades in early December, inspired by Krampus, the Central European folk figure who threatens naughty children into being good just in time for the visit of Saint Nicholas on 6 December. The video opens with an exasperated mother shouting at her pillow-fighting children to be good because "Krampus is watching!" Next, a woman holding a goat "hears" the mother. She metamorphoses into the Queen of the Sisters of Shhh (invented by the krewe as a female counterpart to Krampus, a kind of ice queen who demands silence from rambunctious children), and starts passing their signature snowflake throw from sister to sister, then on to a series of folks who turn into various monsters and Krampuses using cowbells for the transitions. The final Über-Krampus passes a lump of golden coal to a man who becomes Saint Nicholas, wearing a protective mask over his white beard. The words "Be Kind—Take care of each other" float over him before the screen fades to black and "Krampus is Watching" appears. This video has a narrative arc that other #brushchallenge videos lack. When I interviewed him, Krewe captain Michael Esordi explained:

> Part of our whole thing with Krampus is storytelling. I watched a lot of the other videos [...] and sure they were interesting visually, but [...] you could watch it from any point of the loop and it would be the same. I wanted ours to tell a story and tie into who we are as a krewe.

The video plays with light and dark: everyday characters appear in daylight while their gruesome alter ego is shrouded in dark, mirroring their night-time parade. The video also tells a story of the pandemic, by beginning with the children driving their mother crazy in lockdown. And it ends, like the parade with Saint Nicholas, a figure of reassurance after the monsters. The analogy with the pandemic was intentional, as Esordi said. "It's not all doom and gloom, Krampus will take care of the naughty but hey, there's hope, Saint Nicholas is here, [...] this is going to be all right. Be good, and we'll be good".

Another creative initiative was a public Facebook group called Covid Couture, founded by Ashley Charbonnet. It was not tied to a carnival krewe but drew on carnival practices. Stuck at home after her workplace closed, Charbonnet started wearing silly outfits around the house "just to get out of pyjamas", and invited people to post their "quarantine looks" to the group. She set challenges with small cash prizes to create outfits from garbage bags or food packaging, for instance, and made awards ceremony videos to showcase the entries before announcing the winner. Oliver Manhattan, who makes and sells headpieces and costumes for carnival and other holidays, won the "quarantine life" challenge with a coronavirus wig inspired by the famous red-and-grey image of SARS-CoV-2 made by the Centers for Disease Control and Prevention (Giaimo, 2020).

Similar creative endeavours sprang up early in the pandemic worldwide, wherever people had the necessary resources of time and technology (another example was recreating famous paintings, Bruner, 2020). They gave people something to do and a reason to contact their friends. Yet they spread especially well in New Orleans where there were ready-made groups who not only had the know-how to make and perform in costumes, but also the desire to do so and be recognized for it. Costuming and performing are common practices in New Orleans, part of public culture and collective identity. The stay-home mandate imposed new conditions on these practices, but, as Esordi said, "Creative people are going to create". Their creations cheered up makers and audiences. Some conveyed a public health message, explicitly (written messages) or implicitly (characters wearing protective masks). Others – like the Flagettes' video and Manhattan's wig – satirised the situation in a carnivalesque way. The collaboration they required points to another way new-wave carnival krewes responded to the pandemic: finding novel formats for socializing.

Sociability

New-wave carnival krewes are hubs of sociability. People start or join them with friends and make new friends through them, as well as convivial acquaintances. Year-round sociability varies: some krewes hold regular events outside of carnival season, others do not; some friends within krewes might meet weekly while others don't see each other from one carnival to the next. Like the "hidden" amateur musicians studied by Finnegan (2007), krewes are important urban networks that generate the full range of frequency and intensity of social ties.

Once public places had closed under the Stay Home mandate, New Orleanians looked for other, often virtual ways to meet. On six Sundays in March and April, the science-fiction and fantasy themed Intergalactic Krewe of Chewbacchus held a Virtual Cocktail Hour via Zoom, to hang out, check in with each other, and offer help like grocery delivery to anyone who needed it. Only 15–25 of the 2,600 krewe members participated in the two I attended, but they were clearly happy to see each other. Some were in costume; others were stitching protective masks as they swapped news of the unfolding pandemic. Members of the Krewe du Jieux, founded in 1996 as a space for Jewish (emphasis on the "ish") folks to enjoy the very Catholic holiday of Mardi Gras, held their Passover Seder online in 2020 instead of at a member's home. As each household ate its meal, participants took turns to read aloud the Krewe's Haggadah (the text recited at a Seder) from the captain's screen-share. In a similar spiritual vein, the Société des Champs Elysée, a krewe that parades on Twelfth Night, broadcast virtual Sunday services from St Mark's United Methodist Church, where they already provided lunches on Sundays. The Krewe of Krampus held their annual "Krampus in July" membership drive and party online, instead of at a restaurant in the neighbourhood where they parade. Several musicians and dancers who usually perform at the event recorded videos that were mixed with live streams from a few krewe household bubbles. The performers – most of whom were out of work – played for tips or for donations to Feed the Second Line (of which more later).

These online social events were oriented inward, in an effort to sustain the casual social ties that thrive among krewe members. As with pre-Covid in-person gatherings, not everyone participated. Virtual sociability has its limitations: the flattening of sounds that makes background chatter as loud as the main speaker and makes it hard to tell who has spoken, the time lag and screen freeze, the impossibility of side conversations, the ease with which people can leave without saying goodbye. Yet it also has advantages: the novelty of seeing people's homes or virtual backgrounds, the option for faraway friends to join in, the secret multitasking, the low bar for participation (since only one person at a time can speak), the ease with which people can leave without saying goodbye. In these ways, new-wave carnival krewes offered their members valuable moments of sociability at a time of anxiety and isolation. They were also a force for pandemic solidarity.

Solidarity

Carnival may appear to be purely hedonistic, but many carnival krewes build altruism into their activities, donating money, labour, food, or materials to worthy causes. While old-line krewes have the capacity to set up charitable foundations, like the Krewe of Rex's Pro Bono Publico Foundation, new-wave krewes may hesitate between keeping or donating the modest amounts they raise. However, in a country where philanthrocapitalism has edged out state support and a city that has powerful post-Katrina experience of what NGOs and volunteers can achieve (Adams, 2013), the call to "give back" is strong and widely heeded – and the pandemic provided many opportunities to do so, especially as the scale of its economic consequences was revealed. New Orleans' tourism industry all but shut down, leaving thousands of waitstaff, bartenders, cooks, cleaners, guides, performers, and others unemployed. During the three-week period ending 4 April 2020, the Louisiana Workforce Commission pro-cessed 105,000 new unemployment insurance claims in the New Orleans me-tropolitan area (estimated population 1,270,530 in 2019), especially in the Accommodation and Food Services sector (Habans, 2020). In the previous week, ending 14 March, only 1,700 new claims had been submitted in total, state-wide (Bridges, 2020). At $247 a week, Louisiana unemployment insurance is the third lowest in the USA, and though it was supplemented by $600 a week in Federal Pandemic Unemployment Compensation, the latter was scheduled to end on 31 July. In short, many people were going or about to go without, and many others stepped up to help.

New-wave carnival krewes led different types of aid initiatives. Some raised money by selling merchandise: the Art of the Parade Society, an umbrella organization of walking krewes, invited krewes to design print-on-demand protective face masks that members might purchase. A portion of sales went to Meals for Musicians and the New Orleans Musicians' Clinic, raising $2,260 by 18 July. Others donated directly. The board of the Krewe of 'Tit Rɔx ("Petit" or little Rex), which holds a very small-scale carnival parade of floats made of shoeboxes, knew that many of its members, as creative and service sector workers, were short of cash themselves. It gently encouraged donations to Familias Unidas en Acción, which supports Latinx immigrant families (who are ineligible for government assistance if undocumented). Other krewes provided goods and labour directly. The Société des Champs Elysée joined a loose, eclectic food distribution coalition with existing food banks and NGOs, a gay nightclub, a councilmember, restaurateurs, and radical left organizations. Working pragmatically, they served 200–500 meals a week, targeting people who were homeless or immobilised in their homes, who could not access or reheat meals provided by other organizations.

The Krewe of Red Beans was the most visible carnival krewe undertaking solidarity work, due partly to its captain Devin De Wulf's media savvy. Its first initiative was Feed the Frontline NOLA, which paid out-of-work musicians to deliver food purchased from local restaurants to hospital workers. In six weeks, it raised over a million dollars and visited each emergency room and intensive care unit in New Orleans twice a day, distributing 90,000 meals and 10,000 cookie and coffee orders (https://www.kreweofredbeans.org/projects-2). As the first wave of Covid-19 waned, relief efforts shifted from the healthcare frontline to longer-haul poverty relief, and the Krewe of Red Beans launched Feed the Second Line on 24 April 2020. Its mission was "to provide food-love and employment to our culture-bearers – musicians, Mardi Gras Indians, Social Aid & Pleasure Club members, artists, and other cultural figures in the New Orleans community" whose livelihoods and potentially lives were at risk from Covid-19 (Krewe of Red Beans, 2020). Feed the Second Line employed younger, more mobile culture-bearers to buy and deliver groceries, meals, and farmers' market produce to less mobile seniors. By 10 June, they had employed 38 people and were feeding 150 (De Wulf, 2020).

Of course, pandemic relief in New Orleans was not driven exclusively by new-wave carnival krewes; plenty of dedicated anti-poverty NGOs worked on it. However, just as creative responses like Covid Couture emerged through carnival connections and practices, solidarity was facilitated by the social ties forged through carnival. Informal systems of mutual aid emerged, as people found ways to share whatever they had extra – seeds, plants, food, personal care, and cleaning supplies – and posted their pick-up and drop-off points on social media. People circulated information through their carnival networks, which had already established recognition and trust by building casual familiarity.

Some of the initiatives described here might seem like distant "charity" rather than egalitarian "solidarity", especially those mediated by transactions like merchandise sales. However, I still class them as "solidarity", New Orleans is a medium-sized city where the physical and social distance between haves and have-nots is not great. New-wave carnival krewes' members include the comfortable (doctors, professors, lawyers) and the underpaid (chefs, freelancers, artists). From their perspective, the devastation caused by the floods following Hurricane Katrina is in recent memory, the uneven distribution of the benefits of rebuilding is in stark evidence, and the city's dependence on the tourist economy is common knowledge. Although New Orleans has other, less progressive carnival scenes and social milieus, participants in the world of new-wave carnival are arguably especially aware of how precarious people's livelihoods and homes can be. This shared consciousness orients new-wave carnival krewes' Covid-19 relief initiatives toward social justice, while not always mapping out a clear path to achieve it.

Carnival against Covid-19

New-wave carnival krewes' projects of creativity, sociability, and solidarity relieved some of the isolation and insecurity of the first phase of the Covid-19 pandemic in 2020. The three dimensions overlapped: shared creative projects nourished sociability; social connections facilitated solidarity, which forged new social ties; creativity was put to the service of solidarity. The inward-facing creative and sociable initiatives within krewes dropped off as people got used to the "new normal" and meeting places reopened. Other matters demanded their attention in summer 2020: campaigns to defund the police, to reopen schools safely, and to safeguard democratic federal elections. However, several krewes remain involved in solidarity initiatives. For example, Feed the Second Line is going strong at the time of writing (April 2022), and launches new appeals and actions when events like Hurricane Ida in August 2021 create new needs.

I argue that the reason new-wave carnival krewes made a solid springboard for these projects was because they are so tightly woven into the social fabric of New Orleans. Of course, not all krewes nor all members participated. Some people were furloughed and at a loose end, while others buckled under increased workloads and caring responsibilities; not everyone had the time, material resources, or physical or emotional energy for new projects. It was draining for people to process and adjust to the unfolding crisis (especially if they or their loved ones fell sick). A critical dimension of pandemics is that they are beyond individual control and responsibility. As the early goal of "flattening the curve" exemplifies, it is not possible to take full stock of Covid-19 at the level of the individual. Wherever we live, thinking through its spread, its prevention, and its consequences requires us to think at the level of communities and societies. In New Orleans, carnival is already established as a crucial conduit for this reflection. People are used to working together to produce carnival (especially in the new-wave krewes) and they want to celebrate it together, too. They are used to sustaining social relations with a collective bigger than the family or the workplace and more diffuse than a club like an amateur athletics or arts society. New Orleanians well understood that Covid-19 threatened the viability of carnival. Yet carnival gave them extra motivation to tackle the spread and mitigate the consequences of the pandemic.

In fact, carnival became a rallying point in the municipal authority's public health campaigns. Crista Rock, a photographer who works with NOLA Ready, the city's disaster preparedness campaign, managed by the Office of Homeland Security and Emergency Preparedness, took a series of photographs of figures of carnival taking steps to "Prevent the spread of Covid-19".[2] One photograph depicts a Black Masking Indian, Medicine Man of the 9th Ward Black Hatchet tribe, resplendent in his beaded suit and feathers, demonstrating how to "Wear a face covering in public". In another, a Black member of the Pussyfooters women's dance troupe joyfully illustrates the instruction to

"Wash hands often". A further photograph shows a white woman from the Krewe of Merry Antoinettes wearing an 18th-century-style dress with side hoops spreads her arms to "Stay six feet away from others". Finally, a Star Wars Stormtrooper, recognizable in the local context as a member of Chewbacchus, brandishes a can of Lysol to "Disinfect surfaces frequently". All but the Mardi Gras Indian could be seen as part of new-wave carnival. All four do carnival on foot, not on floats; crucially, as performer-participants they are on the same level as spectator-participants. Carnival, perhaps specifically walking carnival, thus helps people make the imaginative leap from the individual to the social that was necessary for tackling Covid-19. As another NOLA Ready poster instructed, using simple pictures, "Wear this [protective] mask now ... so you can wear this [carnival] mask someday". In these ways, an apparently frivolous, hedonistic annual cultural ritual can simultaneously sustain deep solidarity and community connections that are mobilized in times of trouble.

Covid-19 Carnival Coda

New-wave carnival krewes remained concerned about Covid-19 after 2020. Krewe du Vieux and Krewe of 'tit Rǝx were among the first krewes to cancel their 2021 carnival parades, even before the Mayor's Office decided to prohibit them as potential super-spreading events (MacCash & Calder, 2020). New Orleanians found creative ways to celebrate Mardi Gras in 2021, most notably by decorating their houses to look like carnival parade floats as the "Krewe of House Floats", which dispersed the festivities to safe distances (MacCash, 2020). When carnival parades resumed in 2022, Dr Jennifer Avegno, Director of the New Orleans Department of Health, was elected Queen of Krewe du Vieux, an honour the New Orleans native "with roots that go back nine generations" gleefully accepted (Krewe du Vieux, 2022,). However, on January 24, the Krewe announced that Avegno would not be leading the parade on the royal float on 12 February, though she would remain its Queen. Rumours abounded. Maybe Avegno knew something new about Covid-19 risks that everyone else should know too. Maybe the Mayor thought this bawdy, satirical krewe was beneath the dignity of a public official and made Avegno step down.

It turned out that, having recently reimposed the city's mask mandate due to the omicron variant surge, Avegno had received threats against her person credible enough to make her reconsider riding on a throne, on a float, in plain sight. She wrote to the Krewe, "I do not want to create a security risk by my participation, [...] and so believe the best place for me this year is behind the scenes helping to continue protecting our community" (MacCash, 2022). Avegno's gown and scepter took her place, representing her royal role symbolically, if flatly. This coda shows that even socially and culturally embedded community ties are vulnerable, especially during prolonged crises, and that attempts to celebrate and consolidate community can easily be undone by threats of violence. Community is never complete but contingent, emerging through the practices of people who oppose it as well as those who want to belong.

Acknowledgements

This is a condensed and revised version of my article 'Creativity, Sociability, Solidarity: New-Wave Carnival Krewes' Responses to Covid-19 in New Orleans', published in 2021 in *Anthropologica*, 63(1), https://doi.org/10. 18357/anthropologica6312021230. I would like to thank everybody in New Orleans whose insights contributed to this research. I am also grateful to Alastair Parsons for his research assistance, and to Briana Kelly, Brenna Sobanski, and Helen Regis for their comments on drafts. Any remaining errors of fact or interpretation are my own. I received a warm welcome from the New Orleans Center for the Gulf South at Tulane University as a visiting scholar in the first half of 2020. My research is funded by the Social Sciences and Humanities Research Council of Canada. Alastair Parsons' research assistance was funded by the Faculty of Arts and Social Sciences, Dalhousie University.

Notes

1 Videos were posted by the Mermaids of the Sirens of New Orleans (April 16), Sailors of the Sirens of New Orleans (April 19), **Merry Antoinettes** (April 19), **Rolling Elvi** (April 21 and May 16), Lucha Krewe (April 28), Disco Amigos (May 8), Dames de Perlage (April 26), Krewe des Fleurs (May 2), **Krewe of Krampus** (May 18), and **Intergalactic Krewe of Chewbacchus** (May 28).
2 These photos no longer appear on the NOLA Ready website, but were retweeted in its Twitter feed at https://twitter.com/nolaready/status/1265415348263759873.

References

Adams, T.J., & Johnson, C. (2020, April 2020). Austerity is fueling the COVID-19 pandemic in New Orleans, not Mardi Gras culture. *Jacobin*, https://jacobinmag.com/2020/2004/new-orleans-coronavirus-crisis-health-care-privatization.

Adams, V. (2013). *Markets of sorrow, labors of faith: New Orleans in the wake of Katrina.* Duke University Press.

Becker, C. (2013). New Orleans Mardi Gras Indians: mediating racial politics from the backstreets to Main Street. *African Arts*, 46(2), 36–49. 10.1162/AFAR_a_00064

Bridges, T. (2020, March 19). Jobless claims skyrocket as coronavirus spreads through Louisiana's economy. *The Times-Picayune: Web Edition*.

Bruner, R. (2020, April 10). How people imitating masterful paintings launched a sweeping trend from Italy to Iceland. *TIME*, https://time.com/5817117/coronavirus-art-history/.

Clapp, J. (2020, April 12). New Orleans drag flag dancing troupe Flaming Flagettes have a virtual Easter parade in new video. *Gambit*, online. https://www.nola.com/gambit/news/the_latest/article_6a11ccd8-7d02-11ea-a616-e36e63367c3d.html

Dalsgaard, S. (2016). The ethnographic use of Facebook in everyday life. *Anthropological Forum, 26*(1), 96–114. 10.1080/00664677.2016.1148011

De Wulf, D. (2020, June 10). Letter to editor on New Orleans' COVID-19 feeding initiative. *The Lens.* https://thelensnola.org/2020/06/10/letter-to-editor-on-new-orleans-covid-19-feeding-initiative/

Fi Yi Yi, Committee Members of, Breunlin, R., & Ehrenreich, J.D. (2018). *Fire in the hole: the spirit work of Fi Yi Yi and the Mandingo Warriors.* Neighborhood Story Project, University of New Orleans Press, and the Backstreet Cultural Museum.

Finnegan, R.H. (2007). *The hidden musicians: music-making in an English town* (Second ed.). Wesleyan University Press.

Giaimo, C. (2020, April 1, 2020). The spiky blob seen around the world. *New York Times.* https://www.nytimes.com/2020/04/01/health/coronavirus-illustration-cdc.html

Gill, J. (1997). *Lords of misrule: Mardi Gras and the politics of race in New Orleans.* University Press of Mississippi.

Habans, R. (2020). *COVID-19 economic analysis.* The Data Center. https://www.datacenterresearch.org/covid-19-data-and-information/covid-19-economic-analysis/.

Isama, A. (2020, April 7). The real reason the #dontrushchallenge was created. *Teen Vogue.* https://www.teenvogue.com/story/dont-rush-challenge-creator.

Kinser, S. (1990). *Carnival, American style: Mardi Gras at New Orleans and Mobile.* University of Chicago Press.

Krewe du Fool. (2020, April 1). *Krewe du Fool Virtual April Fools Day Parade* [Video]. YouTube. https://youtu.be/-IrDnVpzrsA

Krewe du Vieux. (2022, February 12). A Doctor Playing Queen Playing God(dess). *Le Monde de Merde, 2.* http://kreweduvieux.org/le-monde-de-merde.html

Krewe of Krampus New Orleans. (2020, May 20). *Krewe of Krampus – Don't Rush Challenge* [Video]. https://youtu.be/G5_59YOlOa8

Krewe of Red Beans. (2020, April 23). *Press Release: Krewe of Red Beans, Rouses Markets, the Preservation Hall Foundation, Market Umbrella and the New Orleans Musicians' Clinic & Assistance Foundation to partner for Feed the Second Line program.* https://www.feedthesecondline.org/about

Krewe of the Rolling Elvi. (2020, April 21). *The Merry Antoinettes have challenged us and we gladly accept! [Video].* Facebook. https://www.facebook.com/rollingelvi/videos/557931121501534/

Lipsitz, G. (1988). Mardi Gras Indians: carnival and counter-narrative in Black New Orleans. *Cultural Critique, 10,* 99–121. 10.2307/1354109

Losh, J., & Plyer, A. (2020). *Demographics of New Orleans and early COVID-19 hot spots in the U.S.* The Data Center. https://www.datacenterresearch.org/covid-19-data-and-information/demographic-data/.

MacCash, D. (2020, November 27). Krewe of House Floats, a Mardi Gras 2021 parade alternative, is on a roll. *The Times-Picayune.* https://www.nola.com/entertainment_life/mardi_gras/article_9a3ab472-30d2-11eb-956d-4782c0303e00.html

MacCash, D. (2022, January 24). Jennifer Avegno quits Krewe du Vieux over personal security concerns: 'hatred directed our way'. *The Times-Picayune.* https://www.nola.com/news/article_5c6d208c-7e04-11ec-a460-a7ecfce5106c.html

MacCash, D., & Calder, C. (2020, November 17). No Mardi Gras season parades in New Orleans in 2021; krewes react to 'hard moment'. *The Times-Picayune.* https://www.nola.com/entertainment_life/mardi_gras/article_e5b0dd08-28dc-11eb-b8b2-939bf975bd79.html

Miller, D., & Horst, H.A. (2012). The digital and the human: a prospectus for digital anthropology. In H.A. Horst & D. Miller (Eds.), *Digital anthropology*. Bloomsbury.

Page, J. (2020). *The Flaming Flagettes Easter Virtual Parade 2020* [Video]. Vimeo. https://vimeo.com/406725254

Radice, M. (2020). Doing/undoing/redoing carnival in New Orleans in the time of COVID-19. *Culture*, *14*(1). https://cascacultureblog.wordpress.com/2020/04/20/doing-undoing-redoing-carnival-in-new-orleans-in-the-time-of-covid-19/.

Regis, H.A. (1999). Second Lines, minstrelsy, and the contested landscapes of New Orleans Afro-Creole Festivals. *Cultural Anthropology*, *14*(4), 472–504. 10.1525/can.1999.14.4.472

Roberts, R. (2006). New Orleans Mardi Gras and gender in three krewes: Rex, the truck parades, and Muses. *Western Folklore*, *65*(3), 303–328. 10.2307/25474792

Smith, F. (2013). "Things you'd imagine Zulu tribes to do": The Zulu parade in New Orleans carnival. *African Arts*, *46*(2), 22–35. 10.1162/AFAR_a_00063

Smith, H.P. (2017). *Unveiling the muse: the lost history of gay carnival in New Orleans*. University of Mississippi Press.

Vaz, K.M. (2013). *The "Baby Dolls": breaking the race and gender barriers of the New Orleans Mardi Gras tradition*. Louisiana State University Press.

Wade, L.A., Roberts, R., & de Caro, F. (2019). *Downtown Mardi Gras: new carnival practices in post-Katrina New Orleans*. University Press of Mississippi.

Weinstein, R., & Plyer, A. (2020). *Detailed data sheds new light on racial disparities in COVID-19 deaths*. The Data Center. https://www.datacenterresearch.org/reports_analysis/lack-of-data-obscures-true-levels-of-racial-inequity-in-covid-deaths/.

Willis, R. (2019). Observations online: finding the ethical boundaries of Facebook research. *Research Ethics*, *15*(1), 1–17. 10.1177/1747016117740176

Wolff, T. (2011). *The sons of Tennessee Williams (documentary film)*. New York: First Run Features.

Zeller, M., Gangavarapu, K., Anderson, C., Smither, A.R., Vanchiere, J.A., Rose, R., Snyder, D.J., Dudas, G., Watts, A., Matteson, N.L., Robles-Sikisaka, R., Marshall, M., Feehan, A.K., Sabino-Santos, G., Bell-Kareem, A.R., Hughes, L.D., Alkuzweny, M., Snarski, P., Garcia-Diaz, J., … Andersen, K.G. (2021). Emergence of an early SARS-CoV-2 epidemic in the United States. *Cell*, *184*(19), 4939–4952.e4915. 10.1016/j.cell.2021.07.030

Index

Note: **Bold** page numbers refer to tables and italic page numbers refer to figures

abortion care in crisis 107–116; *see also* feminist abortion accompaniment model of care; accompaniers 115–116; feminist activists support of 108; meeting the demands during pandemic 110–111; as policy issue 112
accompaniers, abortion 115–116
accountability, issue of 126
Achille, Mbembe 27
ACORN 81, 84
action, emotions and 17–18
activists 66
activist strategies, models of care implemented by 108
Aid programmes, in Turkey 150
alcohol-selling venue owners, in Turkey 150
Amphan Cyclone Relief (2020) 99
Ankara Tek Yürek (Ankara One Heart) campaign 152
anxiety, during pandemic 145
Argentina: feminist Green Tide (Marea Verde) 110; pandemic and social movement in 9; poor population in 51
Askida Ekmek (Hanging Bread) campaign 152, 153
Askida Fatura (Hanging Bills) campaign 152
Australia community participation: collection action in settings 68–70, *69*, *70*; during Covid-19 crisis 70–74, *72*, *73*, *74*; Covid-19 restrictions 66–76; introduction 66–68; legal restrictions preventing protest in 2020 67; online and offline collective action in 68, 71; social identification importance 6; spending on Covid-19 148
Australian sample: activists and engaged people in 75; extended EMSICA *74*; extended SIMCA *72*

Avegno, Jennifer 165
"Avoidable Deaths from Covid-19 in Brazil" (Oxfam, 2021) 27–28

behavioural polyphasia, defined 7
benevolent support vs. activist support 147
Brazil access to abortion in 110; effects of Coronavirus in 27–29; representation of Covid-19 3
bubbles 5
Buenos Aires *see also* Argentina
Buenos Aires grassroots movements 51–61; introduction 51–52; online activity of social organisation 52–53; safety and power networks 54–56; social media 56–60; social sensibilities as lens in pandemic 53–54

CAN community kitchens 128
CAN Community Kitchens and a Kitchen Voucher Program (case) 123–124
CAN Involvement in Covid-19 Pandemic Communications Strategy (case) 124–125
CAN kitchen voucher programme 126–127
CANs *see* Community Action Networks (CANs)
Cape Town response to Covid-19 crisis: *CAN Community Kitchens and a Kitchen Voucher Program* (case) 123–124; cases 123–126; challenges of collaboration 126–127; Community Action Networks in 121–122; conclusion 129–130; context and background 120–121; introduction 119–120; relationship building and localism 128–129; research method used 122–123; role of CTT in Covid-19 pandemic 119

Cape Town Together (CTT) 119–120; beginning of 128; widespread participation in 121
care: according to Maria de la Bellacasa 113; contextualising, pandemic in Kolkata and 97–98; definition of 95–96; politics of 103–104
carnival against Covid-19 165–166
CDMX Ayuda Mutua (Mexico City mutual Aid) 18–19, 22
Charbonnet, Ashley 162
charity, notion of 96–97
China community responses: conceptual background and context 38–39; Covid-19 pandemic in 37–38; motivating volunteers 39; professionalisation of volunteers 39–40; results of study 41–47; study conclusion 47–48; study methods 40; volunteering motivation to Combat Covid-19 37–48; volunteering work in 38–39
cinema industry, pandemic and 150
close ties among personal networks, volunteers and 43–44
CMAG *see* Covid-19 mutual aid groups, (CMAG)
cognition, emotions and 17–18
"co-learning" sessions, Community Action Networks and 122
collective action: defined 66; extended social identity model *69, 71, 72*; online, definition of 67; in online and offline settings 67, 68–70; proposed extended encapsulation model for social identity in *70, 71, 73*
collective identity, emotions and 22–23
collective outrage, in offline and online collective action 74
collective work 113
Columbia, abortion in 110
communication networks 54–56
community, Covid-19 volunteers and 43–44
Community Action Networks (CANs) 119–120; *CAN Involvement in Covid-19 Pandemic Communications Strategy* (case) 124–125; in Cape Town, South Africa 121–122; collaboration with EDP and DGMT 124; *EMS Vaxi-Taxi* (case) 125–126; as informal gatherings 128
community kitchen, CAN support of 126
Community-level intelligence, in South Africa 129

community participation: during Covid-19 70–74; experience, volunteers and 85; in Italy and Australia 66–76
community responses to Covid-19 1–9; introduction 1–2; social identities 5–6; social practices 6–9; social representation 2–5
community solidarity, volunteers and 47
conspiracy theories 3
construction of "Us" *vs.* "Them" 22–23
countries, political elites' response to pandemic 19–20
Covid-19 *see also* specific countries
Covid-19, carnival against 165–166
Covid-19 carnival coda 166–167
Covid Couture 162
Covid crisis: mutual aid and 96; and politics of care 95–96
Covid-19 pandemic: as an "economic crisis" 3; average volunteer service hours per day (January-February 2020) *42*; beginning of 4; communities and crisis of 7–8; community participation during 70–74; motivation reported by volunteers 43; political activism and 18–19; restrictions and community participation 66–76; role of emotions in grassroots activism during 19–21; social representation 2–5; social sensibilities as lens in pandemic 53–54; vaccination against 1; volunteer service hours and pandemic progression (January-February 2020) *41*
Crenshaw, Kimberlé 53
CTT *see* Cape Town Together (CTT)
CTT Ways of Working 122

death from Covid-19 6; in Brazil 30, 34; in Mexico City 19; in New Orleans 159; in Rio de Janeiro 27, 28, 30; in United Kingdom 86
de la Bellacasa, Maria Puid 113
Delhi Communal Riot Relief (2020) 99
depression, during pandemic 145
de Souza e Silva, Jailson 34
deviance 8
DGMT *see* DG Murray Trust (DGMT)
DG Murray Trust (DGMT) 123
digital connections, use in Italy 97
direct action, practice of accompaniment as 113–115
"downtown" carnival krewes 157
Dukheimian, definition of religion 3

economic packages during pandemic, in
Turkey 149
economic restrictions 67
economy, in Turkey 147–148
Ecuador, abortion in 110
EDP *see* Western Cape Economic
Development Partnership (EDP)
education level, of volunteers **45**
EMISCA *see* Encapsulation Model of Social
Identity in Collective Action (EMISCA)
emotional and cognitive pathways 76
emotional management, for emotional
work 17
emotion regulation issues, during
pandemic 145
emotions: actions, cognition and 17–18;
collective identity and 22–23; reciprocal
22; of resistance 22; role in grassroots
activism during pandemic 19–21; of
trauma and resistance, political impacts of
21–22
emotions in Mexico City: collective
identity 22–23; Mexico City political
actions and 15–18; political impacts of
trauma and resistance 21–22; role in
grassroots activism during pandemic
19–21
empowerment, feelings of 84
EMS Vaxi-Taxi (case) 125–126
Encapsulation Model of Social Identity in
Collective Action (EMISCA) 66, 69–70,
73, 74
engagement: citizen 39; collective 27;
community, Rogeria and 33;
occupational specialty and volunteering
44; volunteer 38, 42, 43, 44; volunteer
motivation and 41
Engagement aspect, of MOBILISE 146
entertainment venue operators, pandemic
and 150
Esordi, Michael 161
expectations *vs.* insufficiency of assistance,
in Turkey 147–149
extended social identity model of collective
action *69*, 71

favela, Rio de Janeiro's 28, 30, 31, 33, 34
feeling rules: concept of 16; disease and 21;
role in collective identity 22–23
Feminist Abortion Accompaniment Model
of Care 111–116; direct action 113–115;

holistic care 112–113; horizontal power
115–116
feminist activist, support of abortion 108
feminist models, Covid-19 and 108
feminist networking 110, 111
food provision, Community Action
Networks and 121–122
Fumacê, territory of 29, 31, 32, 33
functionalist model of social influence 141

Galindo, María 28
genetic model on social influence 8
government Aid Plans against Covid-19, in
Turkey 145–153
government vaccination programme, in
South Africa 129
grassroot activism, role of emotions during
pandemic 19–21, 24
Green Tide (Marea Verde), feminist 110
Group Area Act of 1950 120
group experiences, facilitating 84–85
Guevara, Ernesto "Che" 55
Guidance on Building Social Service
Volunteer Teams in China 2013-2020 39

Health Promotion Network (RCS) 31
Hochschild, Arlie 16–17
holistic care 112–113
horizontal power 115–116
hotline activists 108
HRV *see* Huerto Roma Verde (HRV)
Huerto Roma Verde (HRV) 19

IBAN *see* international bank account
number (IBAN)
immediacy and salience, Covid-19
volunteers and 42–43
individuals and groups, Covid-19 and 2–3,
5–6, 8–9
"infra-making" 95
infrastructure, during the pandemic 94–95
Instagram 56, 57
international bank account number
(IBAN) 148
"intersectional nature" of discrimination 53
Italian sample: EMISICA *73*; extended
SIMCA *72*
Italy community participation: collection
action in settings 68–70, *69, 70*; during
Covid-19 crisis 70–74, *72, 73, 74*;
Covid-19 in 97; introduction 66–68

Kindness Test survey 79
Kolkata, pandemic infrastructure of care: conclusion 104; contextualising care during pandemic in Kolkata 97–98, *98*; Covid crisis and politics of care 95–96; introduction 93–94; organisational structure of QSYN 98–100; politics of care 103–104; reimagining infrastructure 94–95; resource mobilisation 100–102; solidarity networks 96–97
Krewe du Fool 160
Krewe of Krampus 160–161
Krewe of Red Beans 164
Krewe of Rex's Pro Bono Publico Foundation 163
krewes, new-wave carnival 160, 162, 163–164, 165, 166
"krewe" social club, in New Orleans 157–158
Kropotkin, Peter 133

La Garganta Poderosa (LGP) 52, 54–56, 57–60
Latin and Caribbean Feminist Network of abortion 109
Latin America and Caribbean: abortions and care during Covid-19 pandemic in 109–111; feminist abortion accompaniment model of care 111–116; feminist activists support of abortion 108; introduction to abortion care during crisis 107–109
LGP *see* La Garganta Poderosa (LGP)
localism, Vaxi-Taxi initiative and 128–129
lockdown, in Italy 67
loneliness and isolation, during pandemic 145
Louisiana *see* New Orleans
Louisiana Workforce Commission 163

Madina, Romano 57
Manhattan, Oliver 162
Maradona, Diego 55
marginalised groups, Covid-19 and 8–9
Meetings and events, Covid mutual aid group and 84
Messi, Lionel 55
Mexico city during pandemic *see also* emotions in Mexico city; emotions and collective identity 22–23; emotions and political action 15–18;

findings and highlights 24; grassroots groups organized in 15; method of investigation of experiences 18–19; political impacts of emotions of trauma and resistance 21–22; role of emotions in grassroots activism during 19–21
Mexico City mutual Aid *(CDMX Ayuda Mutua)* 15, 18–19, 22
micro and meso processes, in MOBILISE 146
micro processes, in MOBILISE 146
minorities, Covid-19 and 8–9
mobile vaccination project 125
MOBILISE *see* Model of Belonging, Individual differences, Life experience and Interaction Sustaining Engagement (MOBILISE)
Model of Belonging, Individual differences, Life experience and Interaction Sustaining Engagement (MOBILISE) 145–146
motivation: combating Covid-19 and volunteering 37–48; reported by Covid-19 volunteers 43; volunteer **46**
mutual aid 151; Covid crisis and 96; defined 133; state and capitalism and 96
mutual aid groups description of 151; pandemic in Turkey and formation of 150

Nepal Earthquake Response (2015) 99
"Network professional" volunteers 47
New Orleans carnival and community: carnival against Covid-19 165–166; Covid-19 carnival coda 166–167; Covid-19 in 158–159; creativity in 159–162; introduction 157; researching carnival in 157–158; sociability 162–163; social distance between have and have-nots in 164; solidarity 163–164
new-wave carnival krewes 160, 162, 163–164, 165, 166
non-profit leaders, exemplary quotes form **46**
non-profit organisations (NPOs): combatting pandemics research on helping 38; helping public agencies deploying volunteers 38; interviews with directors of 40; on motivating volunteers 47; reliance and mobilizing volunteers 37, 39
norms, defined 16

occupational specialty, volunteering engagement and 44–445
offline and online collective action 67, 74

political action, emotions and 15–18
political activism, March 2020 and 18
political beliefs or opinions, UK-Covid-19 mutual aid and 140
political impacts, of emotions 21–22
political trust, in Turkey Government Aid plans 146–147
politicisation and polarisation, in Turkey 150
politics of care 103–104
Preventive and Mandatory Social Confinement 51
professionalisation, of volunteers 39–40
"Professors of the Street," in South Africa 129
proposed extended encapsulation model for social identity, in collective action 70, 71, 73
psychological implications, of UK-Covid-19 Mutual Aid Groups 133–142
psychological responses to Government Aid plans against Covid-19, in Turkey 145–153
psychosocial approach, Covid-19 and 1–9
psychosocial view, on political implications of Covid-19 mutual aid 141

QSYN see Quarantined Student-Youth Network (QSYN)
Quarantined Student-Youth Network (QSYN) 93, 94, 97–98, 98; care forms of 103–104; organisational structure of 98–100; resource mobilisation 100, 101, 102, 102

reciprocal emotions 22
Red Compañera 109, 111, 112, 115
relationship building, CMAG participation and 140–141
resilience, during emergencies 38
resistance, emotions of 22
responsibility for community service, volunteers and 43
restrictions, social and economic 67
restrictive measures 67
Rio de Janeiro, corona virus pandemic in see also Brazil; city of 32–33; community actions in 27–28; favelas 28, 30, 31, 33, 34; introduction 27–29; Rogéria Xavier 29–34
Rock, Crista 165

safety and power networks 54–56
salience: immediacy and 42–43; motivation and 39
Santos, Milton 28–29
self-efficacy: coping 139; motivation and 39; volunteers and 43–44
self-managed abortion, defined 107, 112
sense of duty, of volunteers 43
SIMCA see Social Identity Model of Collective Action (SIMCA)
sleep disorders, during pandemic 145
sociability, in New Orleans 162–163
social activism 66
social cohesion, trust and 146–147
"social cure" approach 138
social distance: between have and have-nots 164; and social connection 1–9
social grassroots movements, in Buenos Aires 51–61
social identification: collective action and 68; wellbeing and 83
social identities, psychosocial approach to 5–6
Social Identity Model of Collective Action (SIMCA) 66, 68–70, 71, 72
social implications, of UK-Covid-19 Mutual Aid Groups 133–142
social issues, Brazil and 34–35
social media 56–60
Social media platforms, interaction in 4–5, 9
Social Mobilisation Working Group 125
"social pain" analysis of 53, 61
social practices 6–9
social representation: psychosocial approach to 2–5, 7; social identity and 5–6
social response, to Covid-19 crisis 20
social restrictions 67
social sensibilities 52, 53–54, 56
social support packages during pandemic, in Turkey 149
social ties, volunteers and 43–44
social transformation 146–147
sociological approach, to emotions and political action 15–18
solidarity, in New Orleans 163–164
"Solidarity, not charity," as slogan of UK CMAG 133
solidarity and solidarity groups 97–98
solidarity networks 96–97
South Africa see also Cape Town response to Covid-19 crisis; responses to pandemic 9
Synergies fr Solidarity website 54

territory, concept of 28–29, 32
theory of action 17
trauma, emotions associated with 21
Turkey government aid plans: dynamics of politicisation and polarisation 150; introduction 145–146; lack of governmental responses to the pandemic 147–149; MOBILISE model 145–146; public responses to Government Aid in 151–153; role of political trust in government aid plans 146–147

"ubuntu," principles of 32
UK CMAG *see* UK-Covid-19 Mutual Aid Groups (UK CMAG)
UK-Covid-19 Mutual Aid Groups (UK CMAG): facilitating group experiences 84–85; group experiences 82–84; group scaffolding 81–82; introduction 79–80, 133–134; members of 134–135; mobilisation in March 2020 133; mutual aid groups as "not party political" 137; mutual aid groups within/against 136–137; organised units of mutual aid 135–136; participation and personal impact for members 138–140; prospects for mutual aid groups 85–86; recommendations 86–87; reflections on the politics of 140–142; slogan of 133; sustaining mutual aid groups in 80–81
"Us" *vs.* "them" 22–23

vaccination: campaign in Rio de Janiero 33; against Covid-19 1; mobile vaccination project 125; programme in the United Kingdom 85
Vaxi-Taxi initiative 128
Vaxi-Taxi vaccination 128
Ventura, Zuenir 34
virtual sociability 162–163

("Volunteering Toegether") ZhiYuanHui 39
volunteering work, in china 38–39
volunteers *see also* Quarantined Student-Youth Network (QSYN); community participation experience and 85; coordinators as basic resource to 82; education level of **45**; experience and knowledge **46**; immediacy and salience 42–43; motivation and engagement 39, 42; "Network professional" 47; occupation of **45**; overall trend 41, *41*; professionalisation of 39–40; professional skills of 44–45, **45**, **46**, 47; relationship with other volunteers 83; with relatively apolitical identity 84; in response to pandemic in United Kingdom 79; self-efficacy, community, and social ties 43–44; social skills 44–45, 47; trends, frequency and intensity 41–42, *42*

websites platform 4
wellbeing, Covid mutual aid groups and 81–84, 83, 85
Western Cape Economic Development Partnership (EDP) 124
women, in health care 109–110
World Happiness Report 79
World Health Organisation 2, 4, 58, 108

Xavier, Rogéria 29–34

Zhejiang Province, data collection in 40
Zhejiang volunteers 41, 47
ZhiYuanHui ("Volunteering Toegether") 39
Zhi YuanHui volunteers *42*
ZhongQingYixin 39